The Mediterranean Farmer's Son's Diet

To Mr Vordis
Live Healthy.

2/7/09

The Mediterranean Farmer's Son's Diet

ABDALLAH TAHA, M.D., F.A.C.S.

To order additional copies of this book, contact:
Xlibris Corporation
1-888-795-4274
www.Xlibris.com
Orders@Xlibris.com
49374

CONTENTS

ABDALLAH TAHA, M.D., F.A.C.S.

ABDALLAH TAHA, M.D., F.A.C.S.

General Surgeon

Board Certified, General Surgery, 1983, Recertified 1993

Fellow of the American College of Surgeons since 1984

Graduated from Residency Program in UMDNJ, New Jersey, as a general surgeon, 1979

President, Greenville Hospital in Jersey City, New Jersey, 1992-1993

Chief Section Christ Hospital, Jersey City, New Jersey

Chief Surgeon and Chairman of Surgery (multiple subspecialties) Greenville Hospital, 1996-2003

Director of a Multispecialty Group (seventeen doctors) since 1993, Clifton Medical Center, Clifton, New Jersey 07011

(http://www.thecliftonmedicalcenter.com/)

DEDICATION

I dedicate this book to my hero, my father, who labored his entire life as a farmer to support our family in Palestine. He made sure we always had food on the table and also made education the primary concern for me. My father had hopes and dreams of me becoming a simple physician, and I did everything in my power to make him proud. Little did he know that one day I would become a general surgeon and fellow of the American College of Surgeons, in the United States of America. He died in 1976 due to a stroke that occurred while walking very early in the morning in the cold weather. For reasons out of my control, I couldn't be in touch with him or even attend his funeral. I strongly believe that his life could have been saved if he was under a good doctor care, or had known specific preventative measures for his age group. My dad was never sick, but that doesn't mean he has no sickness, there is a lot of silent diseases, which can kill without warning, one of them is partial blockage of one or both the Carotid Arteries, (the carotids are located in the neck and blockage gives a murmur easy to hear with a stethoscope), the high blood pressure like that morning, (the blood pressure is the highest in the morning when you wake up, drinking coffee and walking or working early in cold weather, both raise the blood pressure more), the high flow of blood in the carotids, can detach a small plaque from the artery(few millimeters), which can give the stroke and even death if there was no body around to help. Any one over fifty years should be taking baby aspirin or another blood thinner if there is no contra indication, and in particular prior to activities in the cold weather., Even if he happened to have a stroke after taking the baby aspirin, or what I GIVE additional SMALL DOSE OF ACE INHIBITOR, (blood pressure pill), he would have had a higher chance of survival. I would like to make preventative actions such as this one common knowledge.

Father, I still ask for your help when I am down. I know you are watching and guiding me along this journey of life. You were selfless, and I thank you for putting your life aside for our family's well-being. You gave me strength; I thank you for the hard-working morale that you have instilled in me. Your honesty and integrity was one of a kind, and I am grateful that you passed these qualities along to me. You made me the man I am today.

APPRECIATION

I would like to thank my loving wife, Taghrid, for standing by me all these years. There were many days when I was so focused on publishing my three books that I did not pay attention to her. However, she still managed to show me love and support. She is a caring mother, a talented artist, and a beautiful wife. I am so proud of her, and I appreciate all the sacrifices she has made in her life to support her family.

I also would like to give my regards to my children, who always were here to lend me a helping hand. I would also like to give my thanks to my cousin Dr. Salah Taha and his wife, Abeer, for their continued support and technical assistance.

Introduction

I believe that there are certain rules and regulations that should be implemented in the United States in order to benefit the well-being of our citizens. America will save billions of dollars by implementing these procedures and concurrently save lives.

I. Chronic smokers (over ten years without any symptoms or less than ten years with symptoms) shall be required to undergo chest x-ray examinations. If the patient visits any doctor and he refuses to undergo a chest x-ray, he shall sign a release form. (This can be compared to the colonoscopy exam that is suggested for patients over fifty).

II. Eye surgery shall not be preformed in a physician's office unless their states give the approval for surgery. Results and complications shall be monitored, just as they are in hospitals and surgical centers.

III. The Carotid Doppler ultrasound shall be performed on all Americans over sixty-five with symptoms of disease, and at any age if it is suggested by a physician. Adherence to this regulation will stop 90 percent of the strokes that occur in this nation. During this examination, a person that is concerned for their health should also undergo an ultrasound that can detect a possible abdominal aortic aneurysm (AAA). This is a relatively unknown silent killer, but it can easily be prevented.

IV. The Dual Energy X-ray Absorptometry (DEXA) Scan shall be executed on women over age forty and men over the age of sixty-five. This x-ray is the most accurate way to diagnose Osteopenia or Osteoporosis. By applying this regulation, our citizens will avoid countless hip, spine, rib, and wrist fractures. A hip fracture alone has 10 to 30 percent death rate in six months after the fracture, this is true even if the patient is healthy and is only suffering from Osteopenia or Osteoporosis.

V. A government-paid-for television broadcasting network shall be created solely for the purpose of informing people of diet, nutrition, and medical news. The station shall be geared to people of all ages. The primary focus should be on the five big health concerns: Diabetes, High blood pressure, Cholesterol, Smoking, and most importantly, Obesity. Obesity is causing our citizens to die young in this country; we should take action to fight this problem now. The television station would give out basic health information such as when to take certain vaccines and when to start cancer screening. Bad habits start at a young age, and we should take preventative measures by educating our children through the broadcast medium which they use the most, the television.

The American Health System
What Is new these days

Hospitals are closing, surgeons and obstetricians are being charged high medical malpractice insurance. HMO's, (health maintenance organizations), are managing the money and not patients health. Some CEOs of HMOs behave like bill gates with a huge salary and stock options—they increase their client's premium of medical insurance by 10 to 23 percent this year and reduce the hospitals' and health professionals' payments. This enlarges the stock price of the company, which in return gives the company the funds it needs to pay the massive salaries to their CEOs. It is almost as if the CEO is inventing new products, but everybody knows that they are indeed not inventors.

I suggest every CEO ought to be a nun or a priest. Hospitals should be managed by nuns who sincerely care about the patients, especially the poor and unfortunate. Eighty percent of the health facilities should be nonprofit run by people with great integrity who desire to serve their community. And those who want to profit from medicine should build their own hospitals (private sector), run it right, and make money from it. Patients who have no time to wait for service, or prefer the upscale private sector hospitals will be the client base for these exclusive medical facilities. Currently, state Medicaid programs are divided into ten companies, each of which has to make a profit. If the state originally didn't pay enough before the establishment of the HMO's how can a company—that thrives on income—pay for the service a medical facility provides? The result is a dog-eat-dog company that does anything in its power to avoid paying medical practitioners for their services. Almost all of the HMO companies are presently trying to prevent physicians from recommending their patients to undergo CT Scans. CT or CAT Scans use special x-ray equipment to produce multiple images of internal organs, bones, soft tissue and blood vessels. They offer much better clarity than other conventional x-ray exams, and are necessary for preventative medical measures.

New Jersey Medicaid pays six dollars for three modalities of physiotherapy (hot packs, nerve stimulation, and ultrasound). The cheapest physiotherapist in New Jersey charges the office fifty dollars per hour, each patient visit cost my office 25 dollars, so what this office does in this case is to refer these patients to the only trauma hospital in the area, they are very busy with emergencies, and physiotherapy is not an emergency, a patient told me they gave him an appointment after one month, I just want to ask a question, is this fair, for this patient to be productive again, he has to be treated now, and not after a month, imagine the stress you will have if this person is your dad or wife'

Congressmen came only to cut the ribbon for the opening ceremony of the new medical facilities that went up in Passaic County, however, they didn't show up when four hospitals closed these past two years. Our political leaders need to wake up and remember emergency cases will die on the way to the hospitals if it is not at a certain range from their homes. It should not be forgotten that if these patients reach the facility alive, they may find the remaining hospital doctors and emergency rooms busy. They may develop complications waiting to be treated, and this is definitely not accepted.

A government implemented law to keep more hospitals open is needed immediately. The hospitals do not have to be trauma centers but they must at the minimum have the capabilities to perform immediate resuscitation and endotracheal intubation. Additionally, the facility must be able to have the means to save bleeding or dehydrated patients until an available ambulance can transport them to the necessary location. And remember that if we have a major disaster, god forbid, these type of cases need a hospital emergency room only, and these emergency rooms should not be far from the accident site, we lost four hospitals in Passaic county in two years, it is so easy to close a hospital, but so difficult to open it again.

What Made Me Write This Book?
Just to Introduce Myself

I am the son of a farmer from the Mediterranean area, who labored all farming duties physically. I used walk to school daily traveling approximately 3.5 miles each way. I became a marathon runner. Our country lacked cars and electricity during my childhood that so we were unable to read or study after the sun went down. My classmates and I would leave every day to school especially early so we could simultaneously read while walking slowly to our designation.

My father worked incredibly hard as a farmer, laboring many hours a day, in our village and in other villages around us located in mountainous areas. Vaccinations were unavailable in Palestine during my childhood. The elderly I knew were born around 1890 and lived to be over eighty years old. They escaped death from infectious diseases and the wars occurring in the region. They received absolutely no medical treatment other than the occasional pill or injection of Nova gin (which can be compared to Tylenol). In the muscle, Novalgin was used for pain; it also can reduce a 105 °F fever in a short time without the use of freezing ice packs. By the way, Tylenol doesn't work till the temperature is lower than 104. Although Novalgin was given to millions of people around the world, it was found to have a rare but deadly side effect (reduce immunity) and was removed from the market.

Those who were born after the 1930s died at the same time as those who were born in 1890. For the reason that by the 1960s, soda, white sugar, ice cream, and sweets flourished and became a dietary staple in my country. In addition to this, stress from wars instigated diabetes to develop into an epidemic. Since Palestine had a poor health system, death at a younger age became commonplace.

I immigrated to this country in December of 1972 as a medical doctor, weighing 164 lbs., and with only 10 dollars in my pocket. I already had two brothers residing in New York at the time of my arrival. In 1979, I graduated from University of Medicine and Dentistry of New Jersey located in Newark, New Jersey, as a general surgeon. I established my private practice in Jersey City, New Jersey. In 1993, I founded a medical center with my two partners, and currently we have seventeen doctors working under our supervision in Clifton, New Jersey.

In 1996, my brother, a hard-working man who suffered from diabetes, developed an acute heart attack. He was taken to a small hospital in Bronx, New York. There he was stabilized and was then he was transferred to a larger hospital that contained a trauma center.

He arrived to that big hospital around 4:00 PM on a Friday. This was the worst time and day to get sick and have an emergency; a lot of doctors already left the hospital for the weekend holiday. It is difficult for surgeons to have assistants. Assistants are numerous, but quality assistants are really hard to find.

My brother was ordered to receive a stenting procedure, which is when metal mesh tube is used to prop open an artery during angioplasty. Everything went wrong with my brother in that hospital; the operation took more hours than expected. He never woke up and developed cardiac arrest few times.

I cried. After discussing his situation with my family and my brother's doctors we had to sign the a 'do not resuscitate order' in case he developed more cardiac arrests.

I lost the man who supported me when I arrived in the USA. With both of my brother's financial and mental assistance, I became a surgeon. I am doing prospering now thanks to their help. It was a sad day—the day I lost him.

My father did not have diabetes and neither did his relatives. My mother also did not have diabetes, but her brother and sister and some of their kids developed diabetes. Hence, the diabetes found in my brother comes from my mother side.

After my brother's death, I felt terrible. I was stressed out (in later chapters I will further discuss the complications of stress), and as a result I packed on the pounds. A routine checkup discovered that I have mild form of diabetes. Immediately I started to watch my diet, but still I had continued to have mild diabetes. I started on Glucophage, the oral anti-diabetic drug of choice for type 2 diabetes.

Diabetes in adults usually starts as insulin resistance, which means instead your fasting blood sugar is less than 100 mg/dl; if it is 125 mg/dl. Most of the time you have high insulin in

the blood at this stage, but it is not working well, and usually the doctors ignore it. You should do the HbA1c, which shows how your sugar was in the past few months, or the sugar meal test (glucose tolerance test) by taking a 100 grams sugar and checking the blood sugar in one or two hours. If your blood is over two hundred, you have diabetes. A diabetic diet is usually enough, but to stop diabetes from progressing, a small dose of Glucophage is a good choice (500 mg). The function of this pill is to sharpen your insulin and make it effective. Exercise, cinnamon, chromium, and vinegar also increase the insulin sensitivity.

So after age fifty-four I developed diabetes, brought by the following, I put weight after my brother's death (caused by stress), age over 40, and family history, these factors combined are a definite cause of this disease. Which need a change in life style in addition to medications to be controlled, or it will control you.

The "Eye Tooth"

My mother always warned me about the "eyetooth". She told me to be careful with tooth number 3—the canine tooth—located on the upper jaw. She said if it ever got infected I would suffer from eye complications. I never took her old wives' tale seriously, after all I was the doctor in the family and I had never heard of anything of that matter. She's gone now, but I wish I could tell her that she was right. Mother always knows best.

A few years back I went to replace a bridge in my left side of the upper jaw. During the drilling, tooth number 3 broke. I painfully felt the drilling in my jawbone. In few days, I developed acute low vision in my left eye the tooth infection had caused dilation and possible blockage in the small veins in the eye. I knew it was related to the infection in the tooth because I felt a streak of lymphatics (lymphangitis)vessels that originated like a thin rope from infected tooth going all the way up to my left eye. It was tender to touch and was painful. The tooth infection had caused dilation and possible blockage in the small veins in the eye. The other place where a lymphatic fluid leak can occur in the legs. That is called lymphatic edema, so I believe I developed edema in the eye from these dilated infected lymphatic's. In the leg type, lymphatic vessels appears as red streaks of vessels under the skin and creates leg pain swelling and edema.

After my discovery I asked numerous dentists if they were aware of the relation between tooth and eye infections. Only one dentist, my good friend Dr. Elsamna, knew the answer. He gave me a picture (shown below) of the face which portrays the way the veins in the face can drain up toward the eye. The canine teeth in particular drain up toward the corresponding eye on the same side. So for the record—eye and tooth infections are related to one another!

From what I know about my case now, it looks like I had early cystoid macular edema, which comes in most diabetics and may not affect the vision, which got worse by this new tooth problem on the left side only (it came from this tooth called canine tooth). I do know from surgery that the face part located above a line extends from the earlobe to the mouth angle drain up toward the eye on each side and down toward the heart.

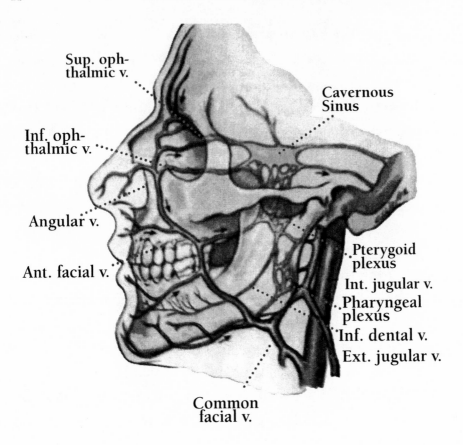

The infected canine tooth drains into the anterior facial vein, toward the neck vein, or in the opposite direction, to the angular (nose) vein, then to the inferior ophthalmic vein and veins around the eye itself, giving the eye infection.

I started antibiotics two days after surgery. I was not told to take any antibiotics and never forget that diabetes and infection do not mix. Anywhere in the body, even an infection under a nail can give abnormally unexplained high sugar and sometimes spread outside the finger to the blood. Diabetics do not get more infection than others, but when they get an infection, they develop more complications, and dentists have to be aware of that.

And if they are good, from the picture of the gum (red, not glistening, and tender to touch), they can tell you, "You better check yourself for diabetes."

At age fifty-eight, I felt the left eye is tired, and its vision is just not like before; it was few days after the tooth drilling was done. By the way, some bridge teeth broke exactly the same tooth I accused of the eye problem, from the metal part, over three years ago, and I never repaired them till recently my son told me, dad, enough you have to fix your teeth, you are a doctor and you have to look good . . . and he added I want to take a picture of you take a picture with a nice smile to be on the cover of this book. I was trying to tell everybody on earth that your teeth are a source of infection, which can affect two important areas in the body:

The heart—it gives valve disease and murmurs.

Eye disease, in particular—it results to infection, which may spread behind the eye and reaches the brain.

Diabetics should start on antibiotics one day before or at least one hour immediately before the teeth operations. Non diabetics should be protected too if warranted.

Vision in my left eye was foggy.

I went to an optometrist looking for help, who referred me to a retina group doctors. I thought I had a refraction problem.

After I went to the retina group, oh my god, my life changed forever.

First, they assigned me to a respectable young retina doctor; he gave me something called focal laser twice in the left eye and once in the right eye, and he said I have cystoid macular edema, worse on the left. When I came back for follow-up, the technician told me, "Do you remember the letters by heart?" I did very well; therefore they told me to come back in six months.

When I went back, they assigned me to a new (older) doctor. I said, "Where is my doctor?" They said, "You were not supposed to see that doctor," and I accepted it. I said in my mind, *The older the better.*

After some tests, their nurse called my office in few days and said the doctor said I need an operation on the right eye. I said I have no problem in the right eye, I had problem in the left eye.

Anyhow, she called back and said it is the right eye. I said I will come and see what is happening. The nurse technician dilated my pupil, took my consent, and sent me to the examination room. This doctor never told me what was wrong with me, what to expect, and what complications I might develop. He switched off the light before he sat on the chair. He never asked me if I have a person to drive me home; then he gave me an anesthesia under my eye, which I did not get in the previous operations. Then he put a magnifying lens with his bare hands and started shooting me in my right eye. During the operation, I saw fire in my eye. I talked and said, "Ah!" He said, "Do you feel pain?" I said, "Yes, during the operation." Apparently, I bled during the operation in the retina, and he cauterized it; but with more laser shots, he was moving as if he was in trouble. Imagine, he burned an area in my retina. I saw the fire, and I felt pain. He said, "Do you feel pain?" I said, "The last part only." I developed a big black area like a root of a tree with other floaters like floating leaves with thin branches in my eye, and I still see these big floaters every single second while I am awake till now, moving five inches in front of my face like a fly.

Next morning after the operation, the right eye went bad; its vision went down, and I couldn't see the TV stock tickers on CNBC. Well, they were blurry for the first time in my life.

But something amazing happened; the left eye improved and came back to help the injured right eye, but I was scared to death. While driving, I keep looking at the cars' plates. My god, I can't see the state name on the plate, but I can see it after I took a decongestant called Dimetapp (OTC), but for few hours then it reversed (it decreased the edema in my eye apparently temporarily).

In two weeks, I went back to the doctor.

The same technician said, "Sign here." I said, "For what?"

He said, "You need another operation." I said, "Are you kidding? Nobody told me I need a second operation." The man almost wanted to beat me up; it looked like he has a reason to threaten me. I said, "I can't see the stock tickers, I am going blind, my vision is foggy. Give me two weeks to improve." He said, "Okay, you will be blind."

In these two weeks, I got worse in the right eye.

I said, "That technician was right, I am going blind, I better do the surgery." Before he started the second operation, I told the doctor, "I see a floater like a root of a tree." He looked in my eye and said it was a coagulated column of protein—in other words, a burned piece of my retina. And he said, "It will go." It never did go; I still see it every time I look at the computer or move my right eye. Straight after the operation was done, he told me, "Amazing, you did not move this time." I knew why. I was desperate for better results. Within six months, I had no improvement. I was in trouble, and then the left eye bled. The treatment is to do nothing, it will clear by itself. My doctor operated me on my left eye while my eye was full of blood; no ophthalmologist agreed with that, and then both eyes now are out.

In six months I deveoped bleeding in the left eye, (called vitreous hemorrhage). It was on a Monday, they said your doctor will be here tomorrow, I said I am bleeding in the left eye, I can't see anything, and I asked what can he do for me, the nurse said he will wait few weeks till the blood absorb, then he will do the retro operation., but my doctor operated on my left eye in two days, and I said to myself if I can't see anything with left eye., how can he see the inside that eye. he must be a genius.

Within days after the surgery, I stopped practicing surgery, lost the chief surgeon position, and the worst thing—I stopped driving. Now I am a prisoner in my own home. I stopped going to friends at night, my two eyes have different visions, and my brain can't calculate the proper distance of stairs, and falls started. I avoided night walks; add to that the glare, which has no treatment except with glasses, good for the daytime. The glare came from the laser when it burned the back capsule of the lenses (a side effect of laser). One more thing, I had edema in my eye (called cystoid macular edema). The doctor looked at it for three years and never saw it. By the way, a doctor told me that in London, any new doctor going for the examination—I am talking about a practicing doctor, one who just finished medical school and not an ophthalmologist—who can't diagnose macular edema, will not pass the exam. In fact, in my training as a surgeon, I was not trained to diagnose macular edema either.

Here I have an ophthalmologist who didn't see it for over three years.

In fact I asked him, "When I did not improve, do you think I have retinal detachment?" He said no. Then I said, "Do you think I have macular edema?" He said no. He told me, "Your vision went down because you lost capillaries." This can happen in retinopathy, but I am sure it is not my case.

I started my own investigations on how to treat myself since he said that I have no macular edema. As a surgeon, I know he burned my retina, and I went badly the next day. This means I have edema mostly in the retina itself, but why does a doctor have to lie? I later discovered he couldn't read my eyes; he just looked inside but couldn't recognize it. In addition, the whole group has no noninvasive test to check for macular edema. Till now I never knew why. A dissatisfied friend of mine, who claims another doctor of the same group blinded one of his eyes, told me that they bought that machine.

I took vitamin E to improve the blood flow in the retina.

Celebrex (anti-inflammatory—it was a hot medicine at that time) worked so good I couldn't believe it. Now it is given for one week only.

I took vitamins A, C, E, selenium, and zinc and cortisone drops 1 percent, which is also high anti-inflammatory and decongestant.

An over-the-counter medicine called Dimetapp helped me temporarily.

All gave me help, but it stopped at a certain level and usually 20/70 on the right eye and 20/80 at the left. Later after more suffering, I found a medicine that can replace all what I took; it is called ginkgo biloba, a pill of 120 mg for a 170-pound person, before I go to sleep. By the morning, I saw it better or equal to all what I have mentioned before, including the cortisone eye injections. I took them for few nights, then I stopped. I usually needed them every time I get a virus or infection. Diabetics don't tolerate infection, and they develop reduced vision after any infection (e.g. teeth and skin infections).

How does ginkgo work?

- It increases the tone in the retina veins, which dilate in retinopathy.
- It decreases the leak in the retina vessels and improves the cystoid macular edema.

This OTC medicine have results like that of cortisone injections, without the cortisone disabling complications. Taking vitamin E, anti-inflammatory pills, antioxidants, calcium, vitamins B1 and 12, and gingkobylopa, can give longer and even better results.

The truth of the matter, I was misled. When the retina doctor told me that I have no macular edema and I'm sure he did not do it on purpose, but you know, it was evident—if he just thought about it. By the way, this busy group doesn't have the simple ultrasound-type test to check on the macular edema. The next two retina consults, I saw have it. In fact, the technician can read it too and can tell the patient the results while he is sitting on the chair during the examination.

When I went to Columbia University, New York, the good doc asked me, "What happened?" I said, "I went for photocoagulation retinopathy operation, and within twenty-four hours. My vision went down and continued to go down." He said, "Oops, that's edema which came from diabetes exaggerated by the operation, and now it is there for more than one year, and called refractory (chronic or not-easy-to-treat) macular edema."

Immediately the same day before the first retina laser surgery, I did surgery without glasses, and now I can't see a black truck in the highway. And I know, since I am a surgeon it is impossible to be from death of capillaries within two weeks the way he said,. Don't forget I am physically the strongest surgeon around. I am very active, and I had muscles since my young age. I know what he says is wrong, but why does he have to lie? I have to believe him.

Let me ask one question. I went to that group with a retinopathy called background nonproliferative retinopathy or mild one, why did they not give me any medicine, checked with any blood test, or told me to start on a diet? And by the way, the second doctor did not know that I am a doctor.

In etinopathy, retina vessels develope microscopic pouches. These come from the inflammation caused by the leaking sugar, the high triglycerides passing in the capillaries, and the fluid that comes with the sugar compressing the capillaries, reducing blood flow, giving weak capillaries, then occluding them. And the body starts manufacturing new capillaries, fast with weal walls, which soon will bleed.

So if they should tell you that control of systemic factors will improve your vision, it is better than their laser at this stage When I saw initially, the retina group, the stage of my disease was called background retinopathy), they suggested no treatment, such as controlling the sugar, strengthening the capillary walls, and giving anti-inflammatory drugs and dilating these vessels to bring more blood to the retina, at least you may postpone the progression of the retina disease. Instead, nothing was done.

Anti-inflammatory drugs, antioxidants, alpha-lipoic acid, bilberry tablets, zinc tablets and vitamins (A, C, and E) as antioxidants are good for prevention in retinopathy. They even didn't think about it

Sugar Control

Treat the high triglycerides. Omega-3, niacin, and olive oil can help raise the good cholesterol and at last, diagnose the cystoid macular edema with a noninvasine machine instead of using your vision—it gives fast a real results.

One thing I want to mention here is this: Before my vision went down, I knew I have two eyes; and after my eye problem, I discovered I have four eyes—two injured and two healthy. The two healthy are my wife's eyes. She is the only person who will drive you, cook for you, feel your pains and not tell the kids, is available at any time if you get nervous—another not mentioned advantage of being married.

Remember what people say: she is the other half, or she is my eyes. Literarily, now, I know why.

In one of my visits, after I started losing my vision after the operation was done, my blood pressure went up. When I went to them the first time, the pressure was 130/70. And I came out with a pressure of 179/90. This is called the stress-type hypertension (white coat hypertension). It usually goes down in one hour or less after you leave the doctor's office.

And in one of my visits, which came to be the last one, this doctor told me, "Doc, I can't do anything more for you. You have to go back to work."

Mama mamita, this doctor is definitely crazy. Either he doesn't believe me or he can't read my eyes. I am a surgeon. I was so loyal to this doctor that I thought he is going to be my lifesaver, Immediately, I felt bad. I felt they think I am not telling the truth.

I told him with a sharp and high voice, "Doc, give me a letter that I can do surgery, And when I go to court for malpractice cases, i I am going to see who will be responsible—me or you (the truth is I told him worse than that)." He said, "No no." I said, "But you can give me a letter to the malpractice insurance so I can do consultation using my low-vision glasses." He wrote, "Dr. Taha can examine patients with magnification." Funny, he just said I can do surgery. By the way, this doctor never told me not to drive, and my vision was 20/100 in his office, more than that they never told me what my vision was that bad, the technician will tell me, the doctor will tell you. But the doctor never told me, I just stopped driving because I can't see well.

The first operation this doctor did on my right eye, was with a different anesthesia from the first doctor I saw, he injected the an aesthetic fluid under my eye, and immediately I felt my right eye bulging, twisted, and I have to close my left eye after I developed double vision.

This group never told me to bring somebody to drive me home. I have to stay in an adjacent IHOP restaurant for a while; then I went to a hotel, and I took dinner while my eye was patched. Now I decided to leave this man.

I went to Columbia University in New York; they diagnosed my problem in minutes, but it did not finish there. I took cortisone injection in my eye. The eye improved but developed eye high pressure (glaucoma). By the way, my wife went to another ophthalmologist, and they dilated her eyes. When she left their office, it was the end of the day. She was driving west, and the sun with dilated eyes does not mix; she was struggling till she reached home. She called her doctor's secretary and told her, you should have told me to bring some body to drive me back home, the glare was so bad that I was scared to have an accident, Please let someone drive, anybody Your doctor dilated his eyes, otherwise, if anything happens, your doctor will be responsible."

By now, I don't trust anybody anymore. If I don't improve, I see the next doctor.

I went to seven doctors, and after four operations and multiple eye injections by other doctors, I got complications. But I was happy since I knew I have good vision, but it kept getting bad. But since I am a doctor, I knew it can be corrected if I'd find the master doctor.

I did find that doctor recommended by a neurologist. I called him the master doctor. He did one operation on each eye, corrected two diseases (glaucoma and cataract) on both eyes, brought me to be able to drive and walk at least in the daytime, and I lived happily after. He brought me back to drive but not to operate. I used to take three medications daily for my eye. One of them can give somnolence, and you can go to sleep on your desk, hit the desk with your head because of developing what looks like sleep apnea. The other was toxic pills called Diamox. It can reduce your potassium to a dangerous level, and the eye doctor suggested banana to replace the potassium.

A doctor told me the banana should be the size of a bull's horn taken one, four times a day (He meant banana is not enough here at all with the dose I was getting).

Laser retina complications (not cornea-type laser, it is different).

- Glare, it is disabling.
- Cataract (and with cortisone eye injection), it is blinding.
- Bleeding, immediately and later on.
- Floaters forever—disgusting, humiliating, and blinding.

I developed all the above complications.

- Diabetes may blind you in tens of years; laser can do it in one minute or days and weeks.
- Exaggerated macular edema and when not treated, it becomes refractory macular edema, which is more difficult to treat.

They burn the peripheral vision so you can feed the central vision or the macula and make it better. My doctor killed the peripheral vision and couldn't see the progressive macular edema, giving me no central or peripheral vision.

- Eye doctors know that retina laser is dangerous. Some of them are honest, but beware of the greedy and those with poor training, which is difficult to know.
- How to solve the problem? Laser eye office procedures has to be controlled by the state, and it has to be inspected, results evaluated. It is funny for a surgeon to open an abscess under the skin, clean the skin with antiseptics, drape it with sterile sheets while in the eye they use a lens and stick it on your eye, including the cornea, without even cleaning it. I can't believe it; this group checked my eye pressure with a tonometer made years ago (not the new type with no eye

contact), which was okay. The question is, why don't they buy a plastic cover? Each one hundred costs a few dollars.

- Nobody can do the same in any operating room in a hospital. There is no supervision or rules to cover the office laser surgery. You may say, "Well, a lot of other specialties do it." Sorry, there is a difference.

- The eyes are the only structure in the body which you can see the brain through it. When I got the intraocular cortisone shot, I was told later that if I developed eye infection, if I don't die on the way to the emergency room, I will lose vision in that eye and may get a brain abscess. Eye doctors should not give the intravitreous injections; under-the-conjunctiva injection is safer and has better effect. I was there; I believe this type of injection can be given under the skin of the lower lid. It has the same venous drainage, and it will not infect the eye. I will not mention the exact site so people will not do it on their own.

- In case of laser of the skin or hair removal, the worst you can have are some burns or redness, but you will not have a dangerous complication. But if you have this burn in the eye retina, it is a disaster. Bleeding in the eye is not like bleeding in the skin; a scar in the retina is not a skin scar even if it is in the face. The skin will have no permanent floaters, cataract, glare, and eye infection from the dirty lenses.

- In the operating room of a hospital, there is a nurse who will write what she sees and is well trained and can help the doctor when things go wrong. There is no way a good nurse will accept the use of unsterile objects in the operation; that's why the eye doctors should operate in operating rooms they own because they will fire these good nurses.

- Put it this way: they may give you over two thousand shots with their laser in retinopathy operation (called retro bulbar pan retinopathy coagulation), and don't forget that one single wrong laser shot to your fovea centralis s, which is a little spot in the back of the eye inside the macula, responsible for sharp central vision, the result you will lose your central vision which mean you can't read letters or watch television. It happened in Saudi Arabia by a good ophthalmologist. He told the patient and felt sorry. Do you think my doctor will be brave to feel sorry? When a Columbia University doctor asked for my chart, he was astonished. There has to be a better control on these operating rooms.
- And, patients, please get a second opinion before you do it.
- The eye doctors and most doctors don't know about the benefits of exercise, diet, weight control, vitamins, antioxidants, minerals; and when you go to a retina doctor, he will never check your blood test, triglycerides (very high triglycerides gives a white retina syndrome, and they never call your medical doctor to review your chart. Some just want to do surgery. In fact, they will be waiting to do your surgery. Procedures pay well, and don't forget 90 percent of the retina doctors work on diabetic patients. and they have nothing to do with your disease, They treat your eye as a punctured tire, not as a part of your body.

Diseases including eyes should be treated with diet, exercise, nutrition, and medications; but medications should be reduced in dose with time if possible by following a healthy lifestyle. Most medications, including vitamins and Tylenol, have benefits and complications. So follow my rules to stay healthy and live longer.

Just one more thing.

Does an eye doctor know how to treat high triglycerides?

When it is 1,000 mg/dl, did they ever check on it ever when the normal level is less than 150?

How about telling the patient to bring somebody to take him home before he dilates the eyes of the patient? (Some do ask.) You may say, "Well, they do," Okay, did they ever have the time to tell a patient? I went to seven ophthalmologists, and none of them told me what to eat or control my sugar or even contacted my medical doctor.

Put it this way: if they don't know much about how to treat diseases causing the eye problem, they should learn now.

And if they know, tell them, "Please open your mouth and help the unfortunate doc."

Aging Is a Negative Factor

Every year our systolic blood pressure goes up one point.

Every year we lose 1 percent of our muscles.

Every year we replace the 1 percent lost muscle with fat.

Every year we lose 1 percent of our brain nerve cells (originally one hundred billion).

Every year we lose 1 percent of our pancreatic insulin-secreting cells (originally one million); these cells are present in the center of five thousand islets in the pancreas. Loss of 40 to 60 percent of these cells gives diabetes.

Maximum breathing capacity decreases 1 percent per year, and cardiovascular function decreases 1 percent per year.

Our reflexes or the speed in which our impulses travel in the nerves is reduced 1 percent per year.

Moving bowel less than once per day can increase inflammation by removing toxins and food end products.

To improve all of the above, mind the following:

- Exercise (you put muscles, lose fat, increase metabolic rate, improve reflexes and balance, sharpen the insulin, lower the cholesterol, and reduce stress).
- Avoid too much sugar to reduce over function of the insulin-secreting cells, I mean beating the pancreas.
- Antioxidants or anti-free radicals. Sage, rosemary, and *Zaater* to keep the neurotransmitters in the brain functioning.
- Use it or lose your brain. I mean play cards, play the stocks (usually you will lose money, but you keep the brain excited, so use a small amount please, go to the church and get involved, help the poor)

CHAPTER 1

Diet

Diet is not a joke; it is a lifetime commitment and not a change in eating habits that lasts for a few weeks. It's important not to diet excessively just because you are going to meet someone and want to look good or because you plan to attend a wedding, and you want to be thin. Looking good is fine, but your health is what matters whether you are young or old. Eating a healthful diet is a lifelong issue, and improving your daily food choices can be the start of a new way of life. A healthful diet includes eating raw foods, foods the way Adam ate them because our genes have not changed much since his time. You can adjust your diet to lose weight, gain weight, or maintain your weight at an acceptable level. I can suggest the best types of food to eat, but I want you to be able to estimate the calories in a portion of food just by looking at it. The portion size that is best for you depends on your age, level of physical activity, the effects of any chronic diseases that you might have, your frame size, your food budget, and whether you are overweight or underweight. Your body mass index (BMI) is your weight in kilograms divided by your size in square meters. The result is a measure of your body fat that is based on your height and weight. To calculate your approximate or what we call normal weight,

- divide your weight in kilograms by your height in square meters (body mass index or BMI),
- multiply your weight in pounds by 703 and divide the result by your height in inches squared,
- or your height in centimeters minus 100 equals your weight in kilograms.

To determine your weight in pounds, multiply your weight in kilograms by 2.25. This method is not accurate for all people, especially weight lifters.

Or find your BMI on the BMI chart.

Body Mass Index (BMI)

Table 1

(Taken from the National Heart Lung and Blood Institute, obesity guidelines).

To use the table, find the appropriate height in the left-hand column labeled Height. Move across to a given weight (in pounds). The number at the top of the column is the BMI at that height and weight. Pounds have been rounded off.

BMI Height (inches)	19	20	21	22	23	24	25	26	27	28	29	30	31	32	33	34	35
							Body Weight (pounds)										
58	91	96	100	105	110	115	119	124	129	134	138	143	148	153	158	162	167
59	94	99	104	109	114	119	124	128	133	138	143	148	153	158	163	168	173
60	97	102	107	112	118	123	128	133	138	143	148	153	158	163	168	174	179
61	100	106	111	116	122	127	132	137	143	148	153	158	164	169	174	180	185
62	104	109	115	120	126	131	136	142	147	153	158	164	169	175	180	186	191
63	107	113	118	124	130	135	141	146	152	158	163	169	175	180	186	191	197
64	110	116	122	128	134	140	145	151	157	163	169	174	180	186	192	197	204
65	114	120	126	132	138	144	150	156	162	168	174	180	186	192	198	204	210
66	118	124	130	136	142	148	155	161	167	173	179	186	192	198	204	210	216
67	121	127	134	140	146	153	159	166	172	178	185	191	198	204	211	217	223
68	125	131	138	144	151	158	164	171	177	184	190	197	203	210	216	223	230
69	128	135	142	149	155	162	169	176	182	189	196	203	209	216	223	230	236
70	132	139	146	153	160	167	174	181	188	195	202	209	216	222	229	236	243
71	136	143	150	157	165	172	179	186	193	200	208	215	222	229	236	243	250
72	140	147	154	162	169	177	184	191	199	206	213	221	228	235	242	250	258
73	144	151	159	166	174	182	189	197	204	212	219	227	235	242	250	257	265
74	148	155	163	171	179	186	194	202	210	218	225	233	241	249	256	264	272
75	152	160	168	176	184	192	200	208	216	224	232	240	248	256	264	272	279
76	156	164	172	180	189	197	205	213	221	230	238	246	254	263	271	279	287

Continuation, Table 2

To use the table, find the appropriate height in the left-hand column labeled Height. Move across to a given weight. The number at the top of the column is the BMI at that height and weight. Pounds have been rounded off.

BMI Height (inches)	36	37	38	39	40	41	42	43	44	45	46	47	48	49	50	51	52	53	54
								Body Weight (pounds)											
58	172	177	181	186	191	196	201	205	210	215	220	224	229	234	239	244	248	253	258
59	178	183	188	193	198	203	208	212	217	222	227	232	237	242	247	252	257	262	267
60	184	189	194	199	204	209	215	220	225	230	235	240	245	250	255	261	266	271	276
61	190	195	201	206	211	217	222	227	232	238	243	248	254	259	264	269	275	280	285
62	196	202	207	213	218	224	229	235	240	246	251	256	262	267	273	278	284	289	295
63	203	208	214	220	225	231	237	242	248	254	259	265	270	278	282	287	293	299	304
64	209	215	221	227	232	238	244	250	256	262	267	273	279	285	291	296	302	308	314
65	216	222	228	234	240	246	252	258	264	270	276	282	288	294	300	306	312	318	324
66	223	229	235	241	247	253	260	266	272	278	284	291	297	303	309	315	322	328	334
67	230	236	242	249	255	261	268	274	280	287	293	299	306	312	319	325	331	338	344
68	236	243	249	256	262	269	276	282	289	295	302	308	315	322	328	335	341	348	354

This type of chart is for people who know what the BMI is. It is good for health professionals and, in particular, nutritionists. By the way, it doesn't give the right picture for muscular people such as wrestlers. Most of my patients want to know how much weight to lose. To be more healthy, for these type of patients, I suggest the MetLife insurance table.

MetLife Height and Weight Tables
Men

Height Feet	Inches	Small Frame	Medium Frame	Large Frame
5	2	128-134	131-141	138-150
5	3	130-136	133-143	140-153
5	4	132-138	136-145	142-156
5	5	134-140	137-148	144-160
5	6	136-142	139-151	146-164
5	7	138-145	142-154	149-168
5	8	140-148	145-157	152-172
5	9	142-151	148-160	155-176
5	11	144-154	151-163	158-180
6	0	149-160	157-170	164-188s
6	1	152-164	160-174	168-192
6	2	155-168	164-178	172-197
6	3	158-172	167-182	176-202
6	4	162-176	171-187	181-207

Women

Height Feet Inches	Small Frame	Medium Frame	Large Frame
4 10	102-111	109-121	118-131
4 11	103-113	111-123	120-134
5 0	104-115	113-126	122-137
5 1	106-118	115-129	125-140
5 2	108-121	118-132	128-143
5 3	111-124	121-135	131-147
5 4	114-127	124-138	134-151
5	117-130	127-141	137-155
5 6	120-133	130-144	140-159
5 7	123-136	133-147	143-163
5 8	126-139	136-150	145-167
5 9	129-142	139-153	149-170
5 10	132-145	142-156	152-173
5 11	135-148	145-159	155-176
6 0	138-151	148-162	158-179

Remember the following:

- A BMI lower than 18 shows that you are underweight, which can be as harmful to your health as being overweight.
- A BMI of 18 to 24.99 is acceptable and indicates a weight within the normal range.
- A BMI of 25 to 29.99 indicates overweight, which is a risk factor for many diseases.
- A BMI of 30 to 40 shows that you are obese and prone to the development of many chronic diseases. You need treatment to lose weight.
- A BMI that is higher than 40 shows that you are extremely obese, which is a dangerous condition. Seek help as soon as possible—I mean today!

Research has shown that a BMI higher than 26 is associated with some chronic diseases and that the higher the BMI, the more severe those diseases are. Diabetes, hypertension, and cardiovascular diseases are the disorders most often associated with overweight and obesity; but the incidence of back and knee pains, lung diseases, and some cancers is higher in those who are overweight or obese than in people whose weight is within normal limits.

As a measurement of body mass, the BMI scale applies to most people with the exception of athletes or bodybuilders with well-developed muscles, in whom a high BMI is not a sign for concern. Most insurance companies would like you to have a BMI that is slightly higher than 19, in case you must undergo surgery and cannot eat for a few days. I agree with that recommendation.

Waist-to-Hip Ratio

More important than the BMI is the waist-to-hip ratio, which indicates the sites at which fat is primarily stored in the body rather than just the amount of stored fat. The waist-to-hip ratio is the circumference of the belly divided by the hip circumference. If the waist-to-hip ratio is greater than 0.85 in men and 0.76 in women, then it is high. Research has shown that people who have a pear shape (in which fat is stored around the hips) experience fewer health problems such as cardiovascular diseases than people with apple-shaped body.

Overweight

Let's examine the effects of being overweight, which most of us are. If you have diabetes and are overweight, losing 7 percent of your weight is better than any medication you take. If you do not have diabetes and you lose excess weight, you can reduce your risk of becoming diabetic. If you have diabetes and you lose extra pounds, you can reduce the severity of your diabetes, you can decrease the medications you take by half, and in some cases, you may not require inject able insulin and can convert your treatment to an oral medication, which is easier to manage. If you are overweight, regardless of whether you have diabetes, losing excess weight can reduce your risk for cardiovascular disease, the effects of arthritis, your overall risk for illness, and your levels of bad cholesterol. Remember that maintaining a healthful weight is a life extender, and that being overweight is like carrying a bag weighing twelve to fifteen pounds on your back. Your heart has to feed that Bag and your joints must support its weight.

Sometimes, following a healthful diet to ensure that you maintain an appropriate weight involves a change in lifestyle and/or a change in the contents of your refrigerator and the number of meals and snacks that you consume each day. As you decide which food choices are best for you, here are some helpful points to remember.

- Do not eat just one type of food. Eat five to seven types in small amounts at a time.
- Eat fruits and vegetables raw when possible.
- Become familiar with food values so that you can estimate the calories in a portion of food just by looking at it.
- Vegetables are low in calories, so eat one or two cups at a time.
- Fruits and beans contain a moderate number of calories per cup, so eat a maximum of one-half cup at a time.
- Eat white bread in small portions.
- Eat very lean grilled meat, up to 3.5 oz., with minimal carbohydrate (a half slice of bread), vegetables, and leafy

green salad. It is good for weight control and satiety and is tolerated by diabetics.

- Eat ice cream and sugary foods, which are high in calories, in minimal amounts that are just enough to satisfy your cravings.

- Eating too many extra carbohydrates and too much fat will increase your weight because the extra sugar consumed will be stored as glycogen in your muscles. The body can store enough sugar for one day's supply in the liver; and the extra sugar that is consumed is deposited as fat in the muscles, liver, belly, and under the skin.

- A high-fat diet alone does not cause overweight because the human body is a fat-burning machine.

- Engaging in strenuous exercises prevents or limits weight gain if you consume a moderate amount of carbohydrates and fat each day. The amount of food that you eat is important, but exercise can prevent or reverse weight gain. For example, a male teacher who is five feet six inches tall, has a large frame, and doesn't exercise needs 1,800 calories per day. A similar person who works in a construction needs 3,000 or more calories daily. Your job and level of physical activity determine the number of calories that you need each day. We gain weight when we consume more calories than we burn. To lose 1 pound of fat, you must burn 3,500 calories or 500 extra calories per day for one week. If you consume 1,800 calories per day, you must burn 2,300 calories per day.

Types of Work

- Light or sedentary spends one hundred calories per hour— teachers, desk workers, and computer operators.

- Medium spends up to four hundred calories per hour—walking, gardening, collecting fruits from trees, and playing tennis.
- Heavy spends five hundred to nine hundred calories per hour)—construction work.

To burn four hundred extra calories per day, you must engage in the following activities:

- 1 hour of aerobic exercise
- 1 hour of gardening or cutting grass
- 1 hour of playing basketball
- 1 hour of hiking or biking
- 1 hour of walking at a rate of four miles per hour

Just remember, calorie expenditure depends on the type of the exercise as well as your weight. For example, if you weigh 200 lb, your hourly calorie expenditure is the following:

- Sitting—90 cal
- Sitting and playing music—120 cal
- Walking—200 cal
- Walking fast—350 cal
- Running a marathoner—750 cal

You can lose weight if you eat a high-protein, low-carbohydrate diet because you will burn fat for energy. However, that type of diet can increase your level of uric acid, and the kidneys neutralize excessive uric acid by leaching minerals stored in the body. If you have gout, you should avoid that type of weight-loss diet as should people with diabetes in whom ketoacidosis, which is dangerous even in those without diabetes, or ketosis can develop.

The liver stores sugar as glycogen. If you don't eat for twenty-four hours, then your stored supply of sugar will have been used, and your body will burn fat for fuel. If the fat is in short supply, then the fasting-hormone glucagon will be secreted, and it will be used by your muscle tissue for fuel. As your muscle mass decreases, you will become weaker. Remember that insulin (the feasting hormone) is secreted when you eat a high-sugar diet, and the extra sugar consumed is deposited as fat. As you starve, however, glucagon (the fasting hormone) begins to act. First it mobilizes the sugar stored in the liver and raises the blood sugar level. In eight to sixteen hours, this sugar is depleted since sugar is essential for the brain cells and red blood cells. And fat can't give sugar, so the glucagon uses the muscle protein to raise the blood sugar.

Glucagon is released into the bloodstream when you fast, when blood sugar level is low, and when you have eaten a high-protein meal that contains few carbohydrates.

Insulin: The Feasting Hormone

The release of insulin, which is sometimes referred to as "the CEO of the body," is stimulated by the ingestion of sugar in a high-carbohydrate meal or by eating a meal that contains carbohydrates and protein. A high level of insulin in the bloodstream can be caused by the following:

- Eating a high-carbohydrate meal
- Genetic factors
- Insulin resistance associated with obesity. Insulin resistance is a condition in which the liver, muscles, and the brain are insensitive to insulin at a normal level. Those three important

organs and their nerve cells use sugar for energy, and if your blood sugar level decreases to less than 35, then seizures and coma will follow. If you eat a high-carbohydrate meal, your body reacts to the sugar ingested by increasing your insulin level. If this sugar cannot be used as fuel within a certain time, then insulin forces that sugar, which is in the form of a fat called *triglyceride,* out of your bloodstream and into your muscles and under your skin; and subsequent obesity, diabetes, or a high level of triglyceride can develop. Insulin thus decreases the level of sugar in your bloodstream, but in response, the brain stimulates your appetite so that you ingest more sugar, and a vicious cycle develops. Weight loss, however, can decrease a high insulin level.

Here are additional facts about insulin:

- It wants to drive sugar into the cells to ensure that fat is stored at all times to protect against starvation.
- It promotes the storage of sugar in the muscles, liver, and brain and directs some stored sugar to be used on demand.
- It promotes the deposit of protein in muscle.
- It causes the deposit of fat in the muscles, under the skin, and around the stomach (abdominal omentum).
- It prevents the breakdown of fat and promotes fat storage, which can result in obesity. If your insulin level is high, then your weight is also high.
- It serves as a fat protector by inhibiting the enzyme lipase, which breaks down stored fat.
- It can increase the levels of bad cholesterol and decrease the level of good cholesterol.
- It increases the level of triglyceride and thus the risk for heart disease.

Weight loss and an increase in your exercise level are the best methods of improving negative metabolic factors. As we said earlier, losing just 7 percent of your body weight is as effective as a medication in managing diabetes and may reduce the dosage and frequency of idiabetic medications by as much as 50 percent.

Glucagon: The Fasting Hormone

If you develop a low blood sugar level as a result of fasting or high blood sugar, the effects of low insulin level or function, either sugar is either not available to the cells as in fasting, or it is available but cannot be used (a condition caused by insulin resistance in diabetes). Because the body needs a continuous supply of fuel for energy, it secretes glucagon.

Here are a few facts about glucagon:

- It converts muscle protein into amino acids to produce energy. This conversion occurs after you have exercised strenuously and your muscles have depleted their stored sugar. Glucagon uses protein from the muscles as a temporary source of fuel. When you eat protein, you rebuild those muscles by using sugar as fuel and protein as the building blocks for cells. That process increases your metabolism for hours after because your body is manufacturing new cells.

Here's some information about factors that influence your good health:

- In people with diabetes, insulin resistance prevents the sugar that is available in the bloodstream from being easily used for energy. As a result, protein, in the form of amino acids, is used for energy. Ketosis, which is the product of a change in the blood pH or acidity develops from protein metabolism. If ketosis is severe, acidosis can develop. Thus, if you have diabetes, avoid strenuous exercise unless you have your medications handy; and one hour before you exercise, you can consume some honey.

- Don't eat before sleeping unless you have low blood sugar.
- Green tea can improve the effects of diabetes, increase metabolism, and improve blood pressure.
- Stress increases weight reduce immunity, heart palpitation, anxiety, memory loss, lack of concentration, and increase the incidence of any disease,

To reduce stress without medications:

1. Walk.
2. Watch late night comedy shows; it is free (Jay Leno and others).
3. Talk.
4. Laugh.
5. Enjoy some stand-up comedy.
6. Play cards.
7. Solve puzzles.
8. Sleep well.
9. Take one day off per week and two days off per month and go to a place where you can't be reached on demand. Period.
10. Exercise.
11. Remember that you are the most important thing around; money is not.

12. Disasters will happen. Manage them and get over them fast.

13. All of us will die, but your loved ones and your family wants you *now*.

14. One day above the ground is better than one hundred years under it.

15. Eating flavorful foods can help you lose weight because flavors produce satiety and send signals to the brain that inhibits overeating.

16. Foods sweetened with sugar tend to increase appetite.

17. Eating too fast can cause you to consume too much at one time and to become overweight.

18. Weight loss makes you feel better and enables you to better control your blood pressure, to reduce your risk for heart disease and diabetes, and to be more active.

19. Weight loss for those who are obese is a treatment that will prolong life and prevent disability.

20. It's sad that people who overeat or smoke often don't change those habits until they are faced with a death sentence like heart disease or lung cancer.

Diets for Good Health

The type of diet that is best for you really depends on your situation. Do you have a chronic disease such as high blood pressure or diabetes? If so, consider these diet tips, and be sure to follow your doctor's recommendations:

- If you have high blood pressure, your diet should be low in sodium, high in potassium, and high in calcium.

- If you have diabetes (and 80 percent of diabetic people have high blood pressure), your diet should be low in sodium, high in potassium, and high in calcium.
- If you have diabetes and advanced kidney disease, your diet should be low in sodium, protein, water, and potassium.
- If you have liver disease and ascites, your diet should be low in fluids, sodium, and protein.
- If you have congestive heart failure, your diet should be low salt in sodium and water.

Glycemic Index (GI) and Glycemic Load (GL)

The glycemic index (GI) is the speed at which carbohydrates enter the bloodstream. Some foods are absorbed quickly, and others are absorbed more slowly. For example, white bread has a GI of 73 and an absorption rate of about twelve calories per minute. Lettuce has a GI of 20 and an absorption rate of two calories per minute. The glycemic load (GL) is the total number of calories absorbed. Sweets have a high GI, but eating a small amount of something sweet supplies a low GL. Some foods produce satiety (a reduced craving for sweets and a desire to eat less). Complex carbohydrates (grains, fruits, beans, and vegetables) have a low GI. Eat those foods in fist-size portions or you can gain weight. The idea is not to stimulate the release of too much insulin, which can cause low blood sugar.

Food Cravings

A lack of vitamins, enzymes, and minerals can cause food cravings as can sleep deprivation, emotional problems, a high level of cortisone caused by stress, or a low level of serotonin. The hormone ghrelin stimulates appetite, and leptin (in Greek means thin, released by the fat tissue) inhibits appetite.

Feeling full (satiety) depends on the weight of food in the stomach; the weight of a full meal tells the brain (hypothalamus, the center for hunger and temperature and energy expenditure) that the stomach is full and no more food is needed. The foods that best provide a feeling of satiety are those high in soluble fiber because they absorb water and their weight then increases. This in turn slows the transit of food in the stomach and intestines. Meat and other proteins, lightweight foods, and liquids produce less satiety. Eating slowly slows calorie absorption and sends hormonal signals of satiety to the brain. Don't keep food near you or around you while you are working, watching TV, or driving because you may tend to eat when you are not hungry.

Don't overeat just because there is plenty of food or because you have paid for a meal. A balanced diet consists of 50 to 60 percent carbohydrates, 25 to 30 percent fats (less than 10 percent saturated fat), and 15 to 20 percent protein.

How Did Farmers Live Before the Luxury Cars and Heavy Machines?

In the rural part of the Mediterranean
They walked to work,
They ran, they talked,
And they worked hard.
They carried things
On the way back,
They played the flute

And danced and sang,
And coming back
They carried food.
And in the dark they prayed and thanked God.
Every now and then
They went to town, walking.
"Walking is good,"
They said.
"It benefits our blood sugar and our muscles,"
They said.
Whole grains
Stone crushed, they ate,
And sometimes whole wheat bread.
"Olives and olive oil are blessed,"
They said.
We planted trees, and we ate their fruit.
We loved the salads and the meat
With all the fat, but only once a week
Or when we were rich, twice a week.
Milk and juice were for the children.
Cheese and yogurt were made at home.
The vegetables we planted, the fruits we loved.
The grapes, every home had grapes and
Plants hanging like drapes
Around the houses.
Under the arbor we sat and played cards and ate grapes.
The black grapes, my dad knew
Are good for you.
I agree; they are good for the heart.
Ask the French; their hearts are fine.

They drink red wine.
Resveratrol. It's in the skin
Of red grapes and black grapes
It is in the flesh of the grape
And in its juice.
The olive oil
We plant the trees
We crush the olives
We eat the virgin oil
We drink this oil
With some bread and cheese
They said it's good,
For the sugar.
It gives no hunger and
You put no weight
We ate potatoes for a treat
Fried in olive oil.
Water was good
And whole grains, but
That was our meal; that's all we ate.
We could eat rice, but
It had a high price,
So we ate it when conditions were nice.
We also ate sweets, but not that often.
Fruits in winter were not there, so
We ate dried figs or raisins.

But now things have changed.
We are rich, and we eat more sweets.
We carry extra sugar in our blood.

We have cars, and we don't walk.
We do not farm, so all of us are teachers now
With a low salary but a car.
We sit in coffee shops and play cards
With a soft drink in hand
The large sweet cola and
We eat sweets and
We smoke.
We are Americanized now.

How many of us are obese now? Farmers work, and they need three thousand calories or more per day. In the Palestine of my youth, those who as infants survived infections (now cured with antibiotics) and epidemics (today prevented by vaccines) usually lived to a very old age (especially farmers, whose primary medication was Tylenol). Illnesses in the village were treated with food and simple remedies, and people who lived to adulthood usually had a long and healthy life.

So let's consider the rules of the farmer's diet. To make it simple, do the following four tips, which starts with the letter *w*:

- Walk uphill, downhill, in the mall, or the park till you sweat. Sweating removes toxins from the stored fat under the skin. And if you can't go out, do it at home as I will show you in a DVD, and make it as a part of life.
- Work can be the best exercise. Plant trees and roses around the house, do construction and heavy road jobs—these are exercise; they reduce stress, improve reflexes and joint mobility

- Watch weight and waist, keep it in check; it is a disease preventor.
- Water, drink eight to ten cups per day—spring water to be on the safe side. Check your city water, and be sure it is safe. Use filters on drinking and shower water. Make water your main fluid intake; it is the safest. Avoid drinks with high-fructose corn syrup and alcohol. Wash very well all fruits and vegetables with filtered water.

Then eat four foods that start with the letter *f*:

- Fiber, it is in the fruits, vegetables, seeds, and beans; it is one of the main parts of the farmer's diet. It lowers cholesterol, reduces colon cancer, and reduces cardiovascular diseases. It is a colon detoxifier.
- Fish, the islanders and Eskimos' life-extender factor (omega-3).
- Fruits, the French life-extender factor. Black and red grapes, it has the resveratrol that is antioxidant and is a dilator of heart arteries; it is like nitroglycerine but without the side effects.
- Fat, but which fat? It is mainly the virgin olive oil, a Mediterranean life-extender factor (the dose of the olive oil is two to four tablespoonful per day) and to replace the meat saturated fats. At the same time, it will reduce the visceral fat and give satiety; it reduces the triglycerides and bad cholesterol. You have to have it in your house, at least add it to salad.

In my country, for breakfast we use good amount of virgin olive oil, thyme (zaatar as powder, a lot of mineral antioxidants, and sesame seeds), whole bread grain (for carbohydrate and fiber) and a piece of cheese (protein and saturated fat), and a cup of tea. Don't tell me it is like eating a cup of cereal with white sugar and a good-size Coke (contains the high-fructose corn syrup). Again, remember fiber, fish, red or black grapes, and olive oil.

Then avoid the next four solid white color foods. They have high glycemic index and glycemic load and raise the sugar in the blood fast.

- No white sugar like that in table sugar, candy, sweets, and ice cream.
- No white bread. Instead, choose whole grain bread, and if you are allergic to whole grain foods, choose barley.
- No white rice. Instead, choose brown rice or unprocessed long grain basmati rice.
- No white potatoes. Instead, eat a small amount of sweet potato in its skin.

So you avoid the high-glycemic foods but also eat the replacements in small amounts (the size of your fist from carbohydrate at a time or less depending on your size).

Proteins

Take grilled very lean meats—grilled skinless white breast chicken and turkey. Goat meat has the lowest fat.

Eat beans in small amounts, quarter to half cup, depending on your size and work. If you can't eat meat to get the complete protein, you have to take grains or rice with it.

Liquids

Take spring water eight to ten cups per day

Fruits, Salads, and Seeds

Eat fruits raw and avoid juice. Serving size will be discussed later. Eat salad and vegetables in large amounts; they have low calories. Eat seeds in small amounts at a time but multiple types; don't forget walnuts and almonds.

Remember the following:

- CoQ10, the most prescribed medicine in Japan; you're brain, heart muscles, and skeletal muscles need it.
- Ginkgo biloba, the most prescribed medicine in France—it opens your arteries, enhances memory, and improves your vein tone, and helps vision in diabetics.
- Avoid the codones, the most prescribed medicine in the USA. It is addictive, increases accidents, and destroys families.
- Avoid alcohol—it has no advantage.

How to replace the four white foods?

- Instead of white sugar, 75 percent of our population can't tolerate excess carbohydrate intake without developing the metabolic syndrome like diabetes. Replacing it by NutraSweet and Aspartame is questionable in particular for memory and for people over age sixty. High-fructose corn syrup is addictive and more toxic than table sugar. Sweet'n Low half pack once a day can be used for coffee when honey is not available.
- If you like your coffee sweet and you are diabetic and even overweight, add honey. One teaspoon of honey contains fifteen calories and has high nutritional value, the same with tea.

- Instead of white rice, take cooked brown rice, maximum the size of your fist, replacing the carbohydrate serving.
- Instead of the white bread, choose the multigrain (not the whole wheat); multigrain has more fibers and nutrition.
- Instead of white potato, including fries. If you have to eat potato, take the sweet potato baked with its skin and the size of half fist—it has fiber.

All diabetics, take sweets in your pocket every time you travel by aeroplane or train; low sugar is a disaster, and aeroplanes may have no food sometimes. Keep it in your pocket and not in your bag. In the bag, walnuts, almonds, peanuts are good. Or take banana or orange in your bag; these foods are sterile, and no need to wash them. Also, keep bottled water in your bag.

Liquids: Juice, Water, and Soft Drinks

Choose water instead of a sweetened soft drink. If you are healthy, consuming one sweetened beverage per day is fine; if you have diabetes, you can drink half a low-sugar beverage daily.

Again, drink water eight to ten cups per day (a cup is 8 oz).

Avoid juice; instead, eat fruit, which contains fiber that slows the absorption of carbohydrates. And remember a cup of orange juice is more than two oranges and contains minimal fiber.

Avoid soft drinks and foods containing high-fructose corn syrup. A 12-ounce soft drink has 120 empty calories; it raises the bad cholesterol; take water with a fruit instead.

If you have to take soft drinks, one with high-fructose corn-syrup drink per day (if you are traveling and there is no other drinks available), keep water in your car with some sweets (if diabetic) or some nuts roasted (almonds and walnuts) if you have no high blood pressure.

Fruits

Fruits have complex carbohydrates, fibers, antioxidants, vitamins, water, and minerals.

Eat fruits in small portions several times (five to seven)a day.

A medium-size apple with its skin. Apples contain pectin, which reduces the levels of bad cholesterol. It has low glycemic factor of eighty calories.

Half a medium-size orange. It has low glycemic factor of forty calories.

Strawberries (up to five at a time). High in fiber, low in calories (the best).

Eat fruits high in fiber so that you consume 25 to 40 grams of fiber daily, such as pears strawberries, figs, and apples.

Eat as much green leafy vegetables and salads as you like. Add a teaspoon of vinegar and a teaspoon of virgin oil to your salad.

Protein and Fat Intake

Reduce your consumption of fats and remove the excess fat from the grilled meat that you eat.

Eat lean animal protein (including fish) in 3 oz portions.

Eat bean protein by the ounce.

Don't forget that beans, fish, and soy are sources of beneficial fats.

Remember the following:

White sugar, white rice, and white bread are processed foods, which means that most, if not all, of the nutrition was removed during processing.

Choose low-fat meat, poultry, milk, and cheese. Eat grilled fish, salmon, and herring, cold seawater-type fish. These have less toxic contaminants.

A high-meat diet is *not* associated with the development of diabetes and obesity. Meat should be eaten no more than twice per week. Buy lean or extralean meat and remove the fat from its edges before you cook and eat it. Avoid fried meat that adds oil to your diet; instead, choose grilled white meat such as poultry. Remove the skin from chicken and turkey before you eat it or choose cold-water fish like salmon, which contains beneficial fats and live in less polluted water.

Opt for low-fat or fat-free cheese and choose skim milk or low-fat yogurt.

Twice weekly, eat fish, tuna or sardines, and skinless white breast chicken.

Boil and eat two egg whites and one egg yolk three times weekly.

Add one teaspoon of fresh olive oil to your salad once to three times daily.

If you must eat in a fast-food restaurant, reduce the calorie count of your meal by removing the bread from your hamburger, drinking a small regular or Diet Coke, choosing a low-calorie salad dressing, and eating just a few fries for their flavor. In doing so, you eliminate 67 percent of the calories from bread and one hundred to two hundred calories in a sweetened Coke one per day. That meal will provide you with protein, carbohydrates, fat, and caffeine but not much vitamins or antioxidants. Most fast-food restaurants now offer Caesar salad, fresh green vegetables, and grilled white chicken.

Spanish restaurants offer pickles (which are fine if you do not have high blood pressure), olives, tomatoes, cucumbers, and flavorful spices, all of which are low in calories and high in nutrition.

Although they are high in calories, juices consumed in moderation are nutritious for children and those who are underweight and athletes. And for diabetics only, if you have signs of low blood sugar, as a main meal, drink a half cup of fruit juice, but remember that juices have the following:

1. High GL
2. Little fiber
3. Poor satiety factor
4. Very high total calorie count

After the age of forty years, the body changes. That is the age of poor absorption. The rate of nerve cell loss increases, metabolism decreases, and the likelihood of having type 2 diabetes, hemorrhoids, cancer, heart disease, constipation, and/or diverticulitis increases. When you reach the age of forty years, you may need to follow the farmer's diet.

Consider the following healthful choices from that food plan:

Foods with a low GI and a low GL—eat them to fill your stomach. They have fibers, vitamins, minerals, and trace elements.

Cucumbers
Romaine lettuce

Half a medium-size tomato
Broccoli
Cauliflower
Carrots
Celery
Spinach
Garlic
Onion

Remember that farmers used olive oil, lemon, and vinegar to season their salads. Olive oil is a life extender; it contains beneficial monosaturated fats and reduces the levels of bad cholesterol. The healthful Mediterranean diet includes the heavy use of olive oil and red grapes. Vinegar has many functions. For example, it increases the absorption of calcium and improves the function of insulin, both of which are important if you want to live a long and healthy life. A salad of lettuce, tomato, onions, sweet peppers, a few pickles, cucumbers, a few olives, and skinless grilled chicken breast that is seasoned with vinegar and little olive oil is a very healthful lunch. If you eat while you are working and you are diabetic, please don't take any medications because your blood sugar level will not increase; and in few hours, you may need to eat a candy to increase your blood sugar level. You will feel full because of the size and weight of the meal and the effects of the vinegar as a satiety factor. You may eat a half slice of whole grain bread too, just to be on the safe side. Let me tell you why: all lettuce salads are low in calories and have a low GL. The teaspoon of olive oil (about 30 calories) does not require the action of insulin to be used as fuel by the body; in fact, it has chromium in it, which controls sugar. Green salads also contain fiber, which slows the transit time from the stomach to the intestines and decreases the absorption of food; magnesium, which enhances the function of insulin; and vitamins. The vinegar used to dress salad increases insulin sensitivity by up to 40 percent. The meat in the salad causes satiety. That type of salad has a low GI and a low GL, produces a feeling of fullness, and stimulates insulin. You could add beans, half a banana, or a medium-size apple to supply complex carbohydrates. If you take warfarin (Coumadin), however, reduce your consumption of leafy green vegetables—some of which contain vitamin K, which causes blood thinning as does Coumadin.

The farmer's diet includes green (unroasted) almonds. Beans (chickpeas, lima beans, fava beans) are often used instead of meat as a source of protein. In Palestine, farmers add cardamom to their coffee; and to their tea they add peppermint, cinnamon, sage (the most popular choice), or rosemary. They usually drink sweetened or unsweetened Turkish coffee with cardamom at night, on holidays, and after a heavy meal to improve digestion. Coffee increases blood pressure by constricting small blood vessels, and it stimulates brain function. Cardamom increases blood flow by dilating small blood vessels, so the vasoconstriction caused by coffee is neutralized by the effects of cardamom. Both coffee and cardamom enhance memory, so beautiful arguments among friends who drink those beverages can continue late into the evening. Tea contains antioxidants and some caffeine, so it is a mild stimulant. It eliminates free radicals, keeps brain cells healthy, and enables greater recall than does cardamom.

Remember that people with diabetes should keep sweets, juices, or sweetened drinks handy when they travel. In Palestine, farmers carry a *melabbas* (a hard candy that is a sugar-coated almond seed).

The sugar in the *melabbas* increases the blood glucose level, and the almond adds magnesium and nutrients removed from the sugar in the candy coating during processing. People with diabetes should eat two candies at a time if they experience the symptoms of low blood sugar.

Today, in the Middle East, you can easily buy a large Starbucks coffee with sugar, as well as most American fast foods. We are Americanized! I ate Kentucky fried chicken at midnight in Amman, Jordan, and people were standing in line. Years ago, most farmers were asleep by that time.

Remember that farmers still eat these healthful foods, which we can also include in our diet:

- Fruits
- Vegetables
- Whole grains at every meal
- Beans every day
- Salad for the evening meal (or salad with bread at other times), which includes the following:

  1. tomato
  2. onion
  3. cucumbers
  4. green peppermint
  5. parsley
  6. olive oil
  7. vinegar
  8. hot fresh peppers on the side

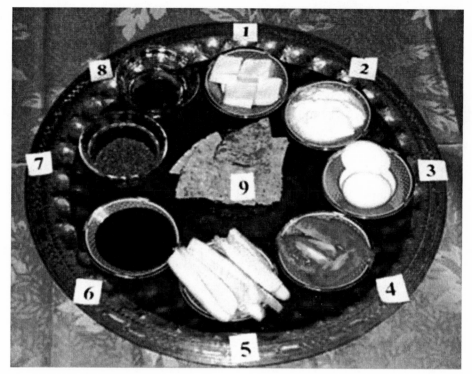

Picture of a breakfast tray with different foods in nine small plates

1. Cheese—source of protein and calcium
2. Yogurt
3. Two boiled eggs—sources of protein and fat Take one egg only or two whites and one yolk.
4. Tomato slices—sources of vitamins, fiber, and lycopene
5. Cucumber slices—sources of vitamins and fibers
6. Black seed paste, for immunity
7. Zaatar (oregano), the antioxidant and the second best antioxidant after royal jelly, a brain memory food
8. Virgin olive oil—for calories and to lower cholesterol. It is a life extender.
9. Whole grain bread, the complex carbohydrate, for brain energy, minerals, and fiber

In most Palestinian villages, breakfast includes these:

- Four-inch diameter, small-size flat plates (four to eight of them). Each has small amount of different food. You don't have to eat everything. All these plates in a big, wide round flat metal tray. And after you eat, the rest is put back in the refrigerator.
- Olive oil (lowers cholesterol) and zaatar (has fifteen times more antioxidants than equal weight red apples) are put in small, three inches wide by two inches deep plates plus one boiled egg, black seed paste (immunity factor), and chickpeas paste (fiber and manganese factor).
- Fava beans paste with olive oil (high fiber, high cal) with whole grain bread, sometimes in homemade cheese. This is the poor man's food, which equals in nutrition to bee pollens and any good restaurant breakfast in the USA with minimal cost, low calories, and high fiber.

In other little plates, they put different foods:

- One boiled egg per person and whole grain bread with olive oil (protein source)
- Olive oil added to salad, chickpeas paste (hummus), or fava beans paste in small amounts
- Halva (ground sesame seeds and sesame oil) that, for people without diabetes, is sweetened

In winter—to give high fat calories and minerals:

- Olives, green or black (has fiber and olive oil)
- Yogurt (*labna*) with or without olive oil added (fat and protein)
- Black seed paste in a small-plate increase (immunity)

- Apple reserves and, if rich, honey in a small plate sometimes (antioxidants and calories)
- Baked potato and french fries fried in olive oil once a week (carbohydrate)
- Cheese divided in half-thumb sizes (protein), homemade
- Milk—regular for kids

In a hotel in Beirut, Lebanon, they give a free breakfast with more than seven small plates and bread. As mentioned, none of them has meat. A farmer's lunch often does not include meat, but it always consists of foods similar to breakfast unless they are working in the field.

They get high-calorie foods—hummus, whole grains, halva, green onion, raw tomato, dried figs, and raisin.

- Whole grain bread with olive oil and zaatar, baked. Like a pizza with cucumber and tomato raw on the side.

The main meal is the supper:

- Squash baked or fried in olive oil
- Cauliflower fried in olive oil
- Cabbage or grape leaves stuffed with rice
- Whole grain couscous (sometimes)

  1. chickpeas as hummus paste, green okra, fava beans, or spinach cooked
  2. grilled meats, poultry, and fish once or twice a week
  3. vegetables, okra, green beans, and salads

In the summer, they eat fruits—anytime of the day—as red grapes, apples, pomegranate, figs, prunes, and berries.

If meat is eaten at a farmer's dinner, it is the main meal, which is usually high in protein. Meat is eaten once a week or when guests visit. These foods are usually also on the menu:

- Rice
- Whole grain bread
- Vegetables
- Beans
- Fruits (especially grapes or raisins)
- Salads
- Turkish coffee, which is high in caffeine, to increase gastric acid and thus aid digestion
- Fish from areas near the sea
- Goat (which is low in fat) and lamb in mountainous areas (both are grass fed)

Do the farmers eat high-calorie diet? Yes, but they use it the same day. Activity is the factor. A seventy-eight-year-old relative of mine who lives in Palestine still walks four miles a day uphill and downhill few times a week after he works in the field for few hours, most days two hours before the sunrise. He was diabetic while living in Bogotá, Colombia. Now he is on no medications, with a heart, brain, memory, and power of a fifty-year-old.

Remember that a high-sugar intake is especially toxic for people of Spanish, Asian, or Middle Eastern descent and for blacks (ethnic and racial groups that together account for 75 percent of the population of the Middle East). These individuals cannot tolerate processed sugar. They are at risk for diabetes, obesity, heart disease, and high blood pressure unless they know what to eat, how many times a day to eat, and how much to eat.

I suggest following these guidelines, which are healthful for all people, regardless of ethnic or racial origin:

- Throughout the day, slowly eat five small meals that have a low GL.
- Don't nibble continuously.
- Learn which foods are healthful and have a low GL so that when you look at the dining table or buffet, you can assemble the meal that is best for you.
- Don't eat if you are not hungry.
- Avoid eating big meals and not exercising or fat will be deposited in your muscles, under your skin, and around your belly.
- Remember that overweight is caused in part by a high-carbohydrate, high-fat diet. When you burn fewer calories than you consume, you gain weight.
- Avoid processed foods, which are low in fiber. As we said earlier, there are two types of fiber: soluble and insoluble. Both types of fiber lower the blood sugar level without stimulating insulin release, decrease the GI, increase the transit time of food through the digestive system, reduce hunger, halt the progression of carotid plaque, and reduce gallstones (which can be caused by rapid weight loss from starvation or excessive dieting). Soluble fiber (like the fiber in apples and oranges) absorbs water, enhances the effect of insulin, produces satiety, improves the lipid profile, and decreases the levels of bad cholesterol. Insoluble fiber (for example, cellulose) is found in nuts, grains, beans, legumes, seeds, fruits, and vegetables. It reduces the levels of bad cholesterol, prevents hemorrhoids and rectal fissures, dilutes

and absorbs toxins, binds carcinogenic bile acids, removes toxins from the body via the colon, protects against colon cancer, relieves constipation, and improves diverticulitis (small balloons in the colon wall that can become infected and ruptured).

- Meat, milk, cheese, and juice contain no fiber.

The Food Pyramid

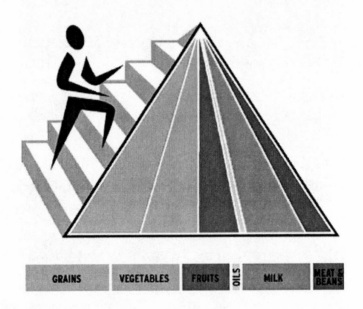

This is the United States Department of Agriculture food pyramid. I'm a doctor. I tried to understand this pyramid; it was not easy that's why I made the food pie to make it easier for people to understand.

❖ The next is my way of thinking to make eating different types of food and easy to understand—the food pie.

First, I made a pie to those who insist on eating the way they eat for long time

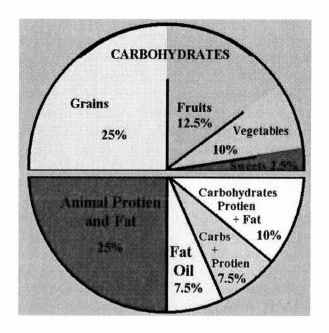

The farmer's son pie, the American style, *improved*

Explanation of the pie

1. Carbohydrate (only) is in grains (whole grain wheat, whole grain pasta, and brown rice), fruits, vegetables, sweets, and soft drinks.
2. Carbohydrate, fat, and protein are present in milk, nuts, and seeds.
3. Fats and oils are olive oil, margarine, canola oil, and butter.

4. Carbohydrates and proteins are in the beans.
5. Fat and protein are in the meat, poultry, eggs, fish, cheese, and yogurt.

Notice these:

Milk has sugar. Cheese has minimal sugar.

Beans are a source of protein with minimal fat and high fibers.

Saturated fats are in the milk products, eggs, and all types of meats, mainly.

This is the overweight and high-cholesterol-people type of diet—usually high-protein, high-fat, and high-carbohydrate diet—if these foods are eaten in excess.

What I tried is to make the pyramid a food pie for a 180 to 200 lb person who needs 2,000 calories per day, is moderately active, and with no disease. Total calorie count from carbohydrate foods is equal to 1,200 calorie per day (equals 300 grams of carbohydrate), 1,000 calorie mainly from carbohydrates. Total fats are 60 grams or 540 calories. Total proteins are 50 grams or 200 calories.

The 2,000 calories needed per day are divided as above:

1. Twenty five percent of calories from grains (whole bread, brown rice, and whole grain pasta), or six servings per day, one serving around 80 calories. For example, one slice of bread or half-cup cooked rice has a total calorie from grains of 25 percent. Also, it can be exchanged with beans.

Twelve and half percent carbohydrates from fruits, four servings per day. Each has 80 calories. One serving equals a medium apple, medium orange, or three-fourth juice. The total calories equals 250 or 12.5 percent of daily needs.

Ten percent from vegetables, seven servings. Each serving has 20 to 50 calories. For example, a cup of green leafy vegetables or three-fourth cup of juice.

Two and half percent from sweets. The least you eat the better.

2. Animal protein and fat. Total calories are 25 percent from protein and fats of fish, poultry, meat, cheese, and yogurt. Each serving of meat is 3 oz with a total two to three servings per day. For example, half a breast of chicken or a medium hamburger. The cheese serving size is 1.5 oz and 8 oz for the yogurt.

3. Carbohydrates and protein (all beans) is 7.5 percent of total calories or 150 calorie. In most European countries, Middle East, and especially poor countries, people eat more beans and less meat. Bread plus beans have all essential proteins needed by the body. Serving size is half to one-third dry beans, cooked.

4. Ten percent from carbohydrate, proteins, and fats (milk, seeds, and nuts) totals to 200 calories. Serving size is one cup of milk or one quart cup of seeds (ten almonds).

5. Seven and one-half percent from olive oil, high omega-3 margarine, and canola oil.

This is the new pie, and it contains all food. I believe it has healthier choices. Some foods are new to Americans (like the brain food as part of your daily meals).

Please tell the bakeries to add sesame seeds to all their grain breads (it has the manganese and vitamin E) or cinnamon to help diabetics, and it is a strong antioxidant. They can also add Turmeric acid (or curcumin) to the bread or sandwiches or the rice (as curry powder)—it reduces Alzheimer's.

Add vinegar to any salad; it sharpens the insulin to use the sugar and good for diabetics.

Use the cardamom in the coffee shops. It reduces the coffee function as a vasoconstrictor to the small vessels under the skin, reducing the temporary increase of blood pressure caused by caffeine.

Tell fast food restaurants to make a sandwich packed with cooked green leafy vegetables with some small pieces of meat (this sandwich can be made of whole grains plus sesame seeds or cinnamon). Tell them to help people survive rather than just eat something. Imagine this vegetable-type sandwich has good amount of fibers, vitamins, minerals, and protein and not white bread, meat, and fat.

Tell them to start using the soybean milk, fortified with calcium, better than half-and-half.

Tell them to use American honey as sweetener rather than the toxic table sugar.

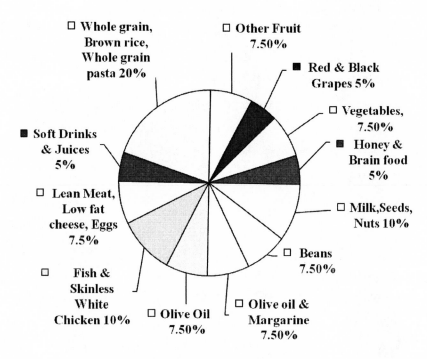

This is the new farmer's son's pie

The Life Extender

Notice the difference between the above pie and the USDA pyramid.

1. Black grapes or red grapes—*insist on it*. Fifteen black or red grapes—50 calories or 2.5 percent—two times a day. The resveratrol factor opens the coronaries. It has more resveratrol than wine with less complications—the French life extender.

2. Instead of sweets and sugar, take honey. One teaspoonful is 15 calories. It has antioxidants and minerals; use it for coffee and tea instead of the toxic table sugar.

3. Double the amount of olive oil, a life extender. As the Mediterranean diet followers, you have to reduce the animal beef fat—take very lean meat. That's why I made olive oil in two places, one of them is to replace the meat fat and the other is to replace the butter and margarine.

4. Eat the cold-sea fish, the Eskimo and islanders' life extender, the omega-3 factor.

5. Soft drinks. One regular 8 oz only. Otherwise diet-type drinks, and it is to best avoid those drinks. Water or green tea with sage, peppermint, or rosemary, it is another memory brain food.

6. The brain food zaatar. It improves the deposit of information in the brain (the intelligence factor). Cardamom reduces Alzheimer's. Curcumin and curry dissolve the beta-amyloid layer in the brain, which forms in Alzheimer's patients. Black seed paste increases the immunity (it works like the immunity drug interferon but without its side effects). Take green or brown tea with sage (the word-recall factor). Or with rosemary (given in weddings thousands of years ago to remember the good occasion). The coffee with cardamom dilates the brain vessels and improves memory or just drink aboya coffee.

One serving of bread equals one slice or half cup of rice.
One serving of vegetable, three-fourth cup of juice, or one cup of green leafy vegetables.
One serving of fruits, a medium apple or a pear (80 calories).
One milk serving, one 8 oz cup of skim milk.
One meat serving, 1 oz or one egg or half cup cooked dry beans.

Total fats is 30 percent of the calories from a 2,000-calorie diet. You need 600 calories firm fat. Six hundred over nine (each gram of fat gives 9 calories) equals 66 grams of total fat. Use olive and other vegetable oils to reduce saturated fats.

I just brought the food pyramid picture here to be familiar with it. You can see that the bands of grains, vegetables, fruits, and milk products are large size while oil and protein bands are skinnier. What I want to do in this book is to show that people's food should be different in their portion and type of food since millions have chronic diseases, and what we eat is an important factor in staying healthy and with less medication. Some can't eat 3.5 oz of meat because they have gout, and others can't eat three cups of milk a day because they have lactose intolerance. Others can't be active thirty minutes per day because they have arthritis or a fracture. My book is for the unhealthy and healthy people. However, this type of pyramid, in my opinion, is for a healthy young adult up to forty years of age, 180 to 200 pounds, with a BMI of 25 to 29.9, no chronic disease, does moderate exercise every two days (like walking for one hour), works eight hours of heavy physical work per day. A person with the same weight and height need more calories but with the same percentage of the types of food. For people with a chronic disease like diabetes, high blood pressure, obesity or people older or younger than forty, a doctor or a nutritionist has to direct you on how much and what to eat. If you are trying to lose weight, you have to eat fewer calories and increase physical activity and remember to eat over 30 grams of fiber-rich food a day.

Consider eating the foods from the food pyramid that are listed below because they have both a low GI and a low GL. Those foods contain 10 calories per serving and about half a gram of fiber; four cups contain the number of calories in a small apple. One serving consists of one cup or a portion the size of your fist. You can eat more of these foods if you are healthy, and they are not contraindicated in your diet:

Romaine lettuce
Eggplant
Cauliflower
Cabbage
Spinach

The following foods have a low GL and contain 3 grams of fiber and fewer than 20 to 30 calories per cup. They are low in calories (20 to 40 calories) and high in fiber.

A medium-size cucumber
A medium-size carrot
A small tomato
A cup of strawberries

These foods have a low GL and contain 3 grams of fiber and 50 to 70 calories per cup:

Broccoli
A medium-size apricot
A medium-size kiwifruit
A medium-size apple

These foods contain 14 grams of fiber and 50 to 70 calories per cup:

> 1 cup of Fiber One cereal
> 1 cup of All-Bran with extra fiber

1 cup cooked beans (lima, garbanzo, fava, black, kidney beans and soybeans) have 10 to 12 grams of fiber but with 230 to 300 calories.

These foods contain 3 grams of fiber and 80 to 100 calories per cup, so eat a half-cup serving:

> Blueberries
> Popcorn
> 1/2 cup of beans
> 1/2 cup of chickpeas
> 1 slice of whole wheat bread

These foods contain 5 to 7 grams of fiber and 150 calories per cup:

> 5 dates (each date is 9 g)
> 5 figs (each medium fig is 55 g, it has 80 percent water)
> a medium-size potato

Underweight people can consume two dates, one-third of a potato, or one fig at a time.

These foods contain 3 to 4 grams of fiber and 200 to 300 calories per cup:

> Brown rice
> Bulgur
> Macaroni

One cup of barley contains more than 350 calories and 30 grams of fiber.

Here are some additional tips. Choose any of the following:

- Skinless, grilled white meat (chicken or turkey)
- Low-fat cheeses
- Skim milk
- Low-fat yogurt
- Olive oil for cooking
- Salads with fat-free dressing or lemon and vinegar
- Spices or lemon instead of table salt
- Diet soda—water is better
- 1 small serving of six almonds, 4 walnuts or other nuts, which are more healthful than a croissant
- 1 fist-size portion of a combination of beans and grains instead of meat
  This complex carbohydrate blend provides good fats and fiber (both of which reduce the levels of bad cholesterol); it is high in vitamin B, iron, and potassium and is low in sodium. It also has a low GL and a low GI.
- 1 medium-size apple
- 1 cup of grapes
- 1 to 2 teaspoons of honey
- ⅓ cup of beans
- 1 cup of skim milk
- ½ cup of yogurt

The following foods have a high GI and a high GL. Avoid them if you have diabetes or are overweight. These are good for non diabetic and underweight individuals.

Bagels
Cornflakes
Potato chips
Doughnuts
Pretzels (not with high blood pressure)

Grains are high in carbohydrates, folate, magnesium, iron, and vitamin B2.

Meats are high in protein, niacin, vitamin B6, and zinc.

Milk is high in riboflavin, vitamin B12, calcium, and phosphate.

The purpose of this chapter is to provide direction for people who have a disease without severe complications. Your doctor must treat your disease and should advise you about your diet. My advice is general; for example, it is helpful for people who want to prevent high blood pressure or for those who are obese and have high blood pressure without renal failure and who need to lose weight. Those individuals would benefit from a diet that is low in salt, fat, and cholesterol. If you eat a low-salt diet, the total amount of sodium chloride that you consume must not exceed 2,400 mg per day. Remember that 80 percent of people with diabetes also have high blood pressure.

These foods are low in sodium (good for anybody):

All fruits (less than 5 mg of sodium per cup)
A medium-size tomato (10 mg per cup)
Large cucumber (6 mg)
Most vegetables (30 mg per cup)

These foods contain less than 100 mg of sodium (good):

> 3.5 oz. of low-sodium cheddar cheese
> 3 oz. of turkey

These foods contain less than 150 mg of sodium:

> 1 slice of whole grain bread
> 1 fried egg
> 1 cup of whole milk
> 1 cup of yogurt
> 3 oz. of shrimp

These foods contain more than 400 mg of sodium (not for high blood pressure):

> 1 oz of American cheese (400 mg)
> 3 oz of tuna (800 mg)
> 1 cup most canned or frozen soups (800 mg)
> 1 cup cottage cheese (900 mg)
> 1 cup tomato juice (650 mg)

For people with high blood pressure, the best diet is one that is low in salt and low in fat and includes the following:

- 5 servings of grains per day (whole grains and brown rice)
- Vegetables, 3 to 5 servings per day
- Fruits, 3 to 5 servings, which are low in sodium and high in potassium
- Unroasted nuts

- A salt substitute
- Dairy products such as
    - ½ oz of low-salt cheese
    - 1 cup of milk
    - ½ cup of low-salt cottage cheese
    - 1 cup of soy milk
- Sweets such as
    - 1 tablespoon of jelly
    - 10 jelly beans
    - 1 12 oz Pepsi
- Low-salt catsup and mustard
- A minimal amount of fat and oil

If you must eat a low-salt diet, then avoid these:

Salted fish
Canned fish
Pretzels
Salted nuts
Salted cheese
Pickles are the worst (which are very high in sodium)

Instead, choose unroasted nuts and seeds, lemon juice vinegar herbs, and spices without salt.

It is difficult to follow a low-salt diet if you dine in restaurants frequently unless you know what you are ordering. When you dine out, try to eat the foods listed above. Don't add table salt to foods and use low-salt, low-fat dressings (be sure to read the food labels). Don't eat preprocessed foods and avoid canned soups unless they are low in sodium.

Here are the daily protein requirements for a healthy person. (Adult, 2,000 calories per day.) 5 oz per day is divided as follows:

2.5 oz of meat
1.5 oz of poultry
0.4 oz of fish
0.3 oz of eggs
0.3 oz of nuts and seeds

You can exchange these amounts, taking more of one in one day and reversing the trend next day.

People who must follow a low-protein diet usually have kidney disease, which is diagnosed with a blood test that shows the levels of creatinine and urea. When it is used to build cells, protein releases urea. Healthy kidneys excrete that urea, but if kidney function is borderline or bad, urea accumulates, and the level of phosphate increases in the bloodstream. Fatigue and low appetite then develop. Meat and dairy products are high in phosphate and can worsen kidney disease. chronic Liver disease and kidney diseases need low protein (less than 40 grams per day), low salt (sodium less than1000 mg per day).

Low salt diet

- Whole grains, one medium slice plus half cup of beans (9 g), which together form a complete protein that contains essential amino acids

- 1/2 cup brown rice (3.5 g)
- 1/2 cup vegetables (2 g)
- 1/2 cup legumes (7 g)
- 2 tablespoonfull unroasted humb-size sweet cheese

Low Salt Diet

Avoid the following:

- Canned and frozen foods
- Salty cheese
- Pretzels
- Salty peanuts and potato chips
- Olives
- Salty salad dressing
- Sausages
- Use of the salt shaker

Low Fluid Intake

The intake will be according to doctor's orders.

We need 1,500 cc per day to replace urine and 1,000 cc to replace water lost in sweating, breathing, and stools. The food usually gives 500 cc per day, so we need 2,000 cc or eight cups of water daily if you have no heart, liver, and kidney disease. Take 2,500 cc per day or more. If working in a hot area, you may need over 3,000 cc water per day.

In low fluid intake, patients follow doctor's orders. Liver cirrhosis, heart, and renal failures.

To calculate fluid intake:

1 cup is 240 cc or 8 oz.
1 liter or 1,000 ml is 4 cups (each cup is 240 ml)

Low-Fat Diet Foods:

Fruits and Vegetables

- High-fiber diet, multigrain's, brown rice, beans, and seeds in reasonable amounts
- Low-fat meats, lean and extra lean; goat meats, the lowest fat in meat; white breast, with no skin; grilled chicken

Avoid High Cholesterol Foods

A 100 g or 3.5 oz of the following foods' cholesterol content:

- Beef brain 1,000 percent of daily value (DV) around 2,000 mg (very high)
- Beef liver, 350 percent of DV, 700 mg (high)
- Egg yolk, 100 percent of DV, 200 mg
- Shrimp, 3.5 oz. 50 percent of DV, 100 mg (medium)
- Lobster, 25 percent of DV, 50 mg (good)
- Lean beef meat or chicken breast, 25 percent of DV
- Skim milk, 1 cup, 1 percent of DV (excellent)

Foods That Decrease Cholesterol

- Pecans, walnuts, soybeans, and pistachio—in moderate amounts
- Tea decreases total cholesterol and reduces the vascular plaques.

- Omega-3 reduces cholesterol and cardiac arrhythmias, decreases triglycerides, and has blood-thinning effect.
- Phytosterol-containing foods like nuts decrease cholesterol.
- In 2004, the FDA agreed that walnuts can reduce cholesterol. Monounsaturated fat in olive oil is the best.

Drinks that increase cholesterol

- Coffee—cafestol, an oil found in coffee, is a potent factor to raise cholesterol. Filter coffee reduce or remove cafestol factor.
- High-fructose corn syrup, used in most soft drinks increases the total and bad cholesterol while reducing the good, happy, or helper cholesterol.

Saturated Fat

Your body needs saturated fat, but remember too much of any food is not good and is usually harmful. If it is meat, coffee, or carbohydrates. Eat it in moderation, (Eat saturated fat but don't eat more than 7 percent of your calorie daily allowance, read the labels, and remember its common source are dairy products and meat.)

There are of different types of fats with different types of fatty acids that are used by the body to produce hormones, energy, and cellular membrane structure. But in excess, they increase the synthesis of the bad and total cholesterol with its bad effects on the cardiovascular system

Common Sources:

- Whole milk—60 percent of its total fat is saturated. It is good for less than four years old, and then after, we need less saturated fats.

- Butter of 50 percent is a high content, but it has the lecithin, which is an antimicrobial and anticancer.
- Beef—40 percent of its fat is saturated.
- Chicken and fish, 30 percent
- Coconut, 92 percent. It has high lauric acid, which improves the immunity and enhances the brain function.
- Palm of 88 percent has 50 percent lauric acid too.
- Cocoa has 83 percent saturated fat.
- Peanut, soy, and corn have 15 percent (good level).
- Olive has 12 percent (good level).
- Sunflower has 10 percent (good level).
- Skim milk has 0.5 percent (very low level).

CHAPTER 2

Exercise (Physical Activity)

Definition of Exercise

Exercise is the activity that involves the use of repetitive physical movements of small or large group of muscles. It can be divided into three types.

1. A healthy person, usually young, with a job eight hours a day, which requires digging, carrying, pulling, or pushing heavy objects to make a living.
2. A planned exercise at home or a gym for a short or long period of time to improve looks, curves, muscle mass strength, weight loss, in addition to heart's health. Again, it is the young and healthy person who has the power and time to do it. Planned exercises are the most available exercises on TV—the target is this age group of people.
3. The controlled, under supervision type like physical therapy at home or in a special medical facility to improve the strength of muscles and prevent atrophy secondary to a nerve, bone, or muscle injury like acute hip and spine fracture. This type of exercise is available in hospitals and special rehab centers.

4. Physical activity for those who are healthy over forty or with a chronic disease like diabetes, obesity, or back pain—healthy but with a less disabling problem like wrist and ankle fracture at any age. And last, those over fifty, with or without a chronic disease. These type of patients care about living a healthy life with stronger muscles and stronger bones to avoid acute disabling fractures, to improve metabolism, improve diabetes, and reduce weight. They have to move to avoid leg swelling, leg vein blockage, and lung emboli. They want to prevent or postpone disabling diseases like heart attacks or strokes. These types of people are busy, have children in college, have many reasons not to go to the gym; they are carrying America on their shoulders. Some of them are the baby boomers. For them and the partially disabled young or old I present my exercise.

How, Why, and When to Exercise

Exercise is a part of life. Jobs such as construction work or office cleaning provide plenty of exercise. Exercise itself can be a way to earn a living (for example, a personal trainer), or it can be a path to a better socioeconomic status like that of a professional athlete or a marathon runner. It can also be just a way to build good health. That is my objective in this book—to help you live a healthy life.

Exercise can help anybody at any age. All of us need exercise; in fact, it should be a way of life. Children should be encouraged to exercise by their family members as well as by their schools, their church and government agencies. Those of us who are poor need access to city swimming pools and parks.

Although everybody needs exercise, each of us must know his or her limits. Factors such as age, size, weight, physical condition, and disease can affect the type and duration of the exercise that you plan to do. My point in this book is that if you haven't exercised before and if you want to be around for your kids and grandchildren, you'd better start exercising. Exercise, like total calorie intake, is one of the most important factors in living a long and healthy life. Here are some facts about various types of exercise.

Aerobic Exercises

Aerobic exercises can be very low impact (swimming), medium impact (walking or dancing), or high impact (jogging or running).

Aerobic exercises have the following effects:

- Strengthen the heart
- Increase cardiac output
- Improve lung function
- Burn calories
- Increase flexibility
- Decrease stress
- Lower high blood pressure
- Build muscle mass

In the elderly it

- decreases stress,
- increases muscle size,
- improves bone mass, and
- improves reflexes and balance.

All these reduce falls or reduce the extent of injury. However, they are not the best exercises for building strength.

Exercises That Build Strength and Muscle

Exercises that build strength and muscle mass like weight lifting improve physical appearance; strengthen bones, tendons, and ligaments; increase tone; and build the strength to perform physically difficult tasks.

Exercise Needs More Energy

If you are 200 lb, you are spending 90 calories per hour. If inactive, like sitting or doing stretching exercises, you double it to 180 calories per hour. Walking or house cleaning and scrubbing walls spend 360 calories per hour. Fast walking and body lifting is at 500 calories; biking vigorously or marathon running is at 750 to 1,000 calories per hour.

Flexibility Exercises

Flexibility exercises such as stretching are an excellent warm-up before physical exertion, but they are healthful for people of all ages, not just those who are young and strong. They reduce muscle strain, improve balance, and can benefit people with certain types of physical limitations, as well as those who are healthy. Flexibility exercises can be performed passively or actively and may require the assistance of a helper.

The Farmer's Son's Exercises

My exercise is suggested for people over forty or less than forty with chronic diabetes or disabling (hip fracture) disease. I have devised the following low-impact, mild-to-moderate aerobic exercises, which can be performed at home to help you build and strengthen muscle, strengthen your bones, tone your body, improve reflexes, balance and decrease the likelihood of fractures or blood clotting, and ensure your mobility for as long as you live. These exercises involve walking a long distance while carrying a weight of, for example five to ten pounds. If you can carry a weight while you are walking, you will mimic the daily activities of farmers, who must often carry heavy objects while they work. However, remember that carrying a weight while walking may not be the right choice of exercise for everyone, especially those with certain health disorders or age older than seventy years. In those individuals, these exercises can cause complications instead of providing help. However, if you do not have health limitations that restrict weight carrying during mild exercise, then the farmer's son's exercises may be the fitness plan for you.

For at least eight hours a day, most farmers perform physically demanding work that is matched by jobs such as construction work. However, most jobs in America today are sedentary, and even children tend to be inactive. The farmer's son's exercises are especially helpful for people whose job requires little physical activity, although active people can benefit as well.

It's possible to perform some type of exercise almost everywhere. You can perform the farmer's son's exercises at home, in the shower, while watching TV, in the morning, afternoon, or night—two hours after meals and three hours before sleep, or before you eat, if you have no diabetes.

You can perform these exercises while

- walking,
- fast walking,
- slow running in well-maintained smooth areas,
- gardening,
- working around the house,
- planting,
- farming,
- marathon running,
- weight lifting, and
- swimming.

Remember, however, that strenuous exercise is not for everybody, especially those with certain types of health problems. For example, if you are fifty years old and have minor arthritis, high-impact aerobic exercise, will increase the likelihood of your developing a degenerative disease in your knees. Brief periods of mild-to-moderate exercise that is performed frequently would be a better choice. If you are either older than fifty years or older than forty years and have any of several diseases such as bone disease, obesity, or diabetes, then mild or moderate exercise that is properly performed in a controlled environment could be beneficial.

Health Benefits from Exercising

Exercise can do the following:

- Prolong or extend life
- Lower high blood pressure
- Decrease the risk for deep venous thrombosis (DVT)
- Decrease the levels of bad cholesterol
- Improve insulin function and the treatment of diabetes
- Increase muscle mass
- Increase metabolism
- Improve joint function
- Alleviate the effects of emotional stress
- Increase strength
- Improve heart function
- Decrease the amount of oxygen needed for cardiac function by increasing the volume of blood pumped by the heart and the volume of blood pumped per beat
- Reduce the heart rate. (The pulse rate of a marathon runner is about sixty beats or fewer per minute, that of a mildly active person who is fifty to sixty years of age is around eighty to eighty-four beats per minute, and that of a physically fit thirty-year-old policeman is around seventy-two beats per minute.)
- Improve balance
- Protect against the harmful effects of smoking
- Benefit both body and mind
- Maintain muscle tone, strength, and bulk
- Decrease the risk for stroke
- Increase insulin sensitivity in people with diabetes
- Reduce the level of blood sugar

- Reduce the levels of fats in the bloodstream
- Relieve the symptoms of arthritis
- Strengthen bone
- Protect against osteoporosis
- Help maintain weight loss by increasing metabolism for a relatively long period after exercise

Remember that exercising appropriately is the least expensive way to stay healthy and extend your life.

Possible Harmful Effects of Exercise

Plaque rupture, which causes some people to die suddenly while jogging or exercising strenuously, can occur when accumulated plaque is dislodged from the blood vessel wall by the rapid blood flow from a vigorously beating heart. If you have a history or a family history of heart disease, you should not exercise strenuously for long periods. Instead, exercise several times daily for short periods. Also, if you have deep thrombophlebitis in your legs, a blood clot that dislodges during exercise can travel to the lungs with serious results. Postpartum cases of phlebitis are also common. Suspect phlebitis of the legs if you notice leg pain and/or swelling when you sit for long periods, such as during air travel. In many cases of phlebitis, a filter that can catch blood clots in the circulation is inserted into the inferior vena cava, which is the main vein that transports the blood from the legs and pelvis to the heart. (Superficial, under-the-skin blood clots give local swelling, under-the-skin bleeding, pain, and later ulcers but no lung blockage. A venous Doppler test has to rule out the deep venous thromboses or DVT.)

Other people who should avoid strenuous exercise include those with systolic blood pressure higher than 160 and diastolic blood pressure higher than 100. If you have uncontrolled blood pressure, do not exercise at all till your blood pressure is well controlled. If you are treated with cortisone or taking ephedra, do not exercise.

Exercise Bulimia

People with this psychiatric disorder are obsessed with exercising, and they over exercise as a consequence. They feel that exercise is more important than work, and they become depressed if they miss a day of their exercise routine. They tend to feel superior to those who are not as devoted to exercising; and although they have minimal body fat, they perceive themselves as being overweight. In fact, some of these individuals seek liposuction to remove imagined fat deposits. Because they exercise for very long periods, dehydration or cardiac disease can develop in people with exercise bulimia. Some people with that disorder tend to abuse cortisone or ephedra and may follow a diet that consists only or primarily of very low-calorie foods. It is important to remember that an excess of anything, even exercise, can be harmful.

Stop exercising if you experience the following:

- Chest pain, even if you think that the pain is caused by gastric reflux or gas
- Shortness of breath
- Dizziness
- Cold sweats
- Irritability

Put it this way: if you can't talk while you are exercising, stop.

Methods of losing weight:

- Starvation
- Reducing your calorie intake
- Eating a high-protein, low-carbohydrate diet
- Reducing your calorie intake and increasing your level of exercise
- Exercising more (Remember that even many hours after exercise, muscles burn calories better than do any other tissues in the body.)
- Weight-loss (bariatric) surgery

Of these methods, starvation is the worst. When you starve, you lose muscle tissue very quickly. After one day of fasting, all the sugar stored in your liver and muscles has been depleted, and your body must use another source of fuel. The fasting-hormone glucagon begins to reduce your metabolism, and you don't lose fat; you lose muscle. You will soon feel the effects of low blood sugar, and constipation develops because you are consuming no fiber.

A slow weight loss of one to two pounds per week (four to five pounds per month) is better. Remember that losing weight is good, but maintaining an appropriate weight is best for good health. Eating a balanced diet that prevents major changes in your blood chemistry levels will help you to feel better while you are losing weight and exercising.

Metabolism decreases after menopause and as a result of aging. For example, if you need 1,800 calories daily when you are twenty-five years old, then you will require 1,600 calories daily when you are fifty years of age. If you are going to exercise three to five days a week and you have disease or a medical disorder, then you should obtain your doctor's approval before you begin your exercise routine.

Start with a low-impact type of exercise or fast walking for a comfortable distance. If you feel good after one week of that routine, then you can increase the length of your exercise program. Take precautions against injuries such as falls. Avoid areas with holes, and try to become familiar with the geography of the area in which you walk for exercise. Eventually (and with your doctor's approval if necessary), you may progress to fast walking or bicycling. If you have diabetes, heart disease, or high blood pressure, do not engage in any strenuous exercise. Even if you are healthy, it is important to know when to stop exercising.

Remember that during exercise, fat is burned for energy and muscle mass is increased. Muscle mass is the weight of your body minus the weight of your bones, fat, blood, and organs. Muscle loss begins after the age of twenty-five years, but if you are active, you may not lose muscle mass after that age; and if you are very active, you can maintain or build muscle mass at any age. When you add muscle, you need fat for energy because sugar does not supply enough energy. For that reason, if you do not want to lose weight or you are a marathon runner, you might eat some honey or extra sugar to be stored in your muscles before you exercise.

Muscular people are perceived by most of us as being physically attractive. They tend to have a low incidence of osteoporosis, they are relatively strong and have toned muscles, and they usually feel healthy. If you are young or middle-aged and you do not exercise, then when you reach the age of seventy years, your muscle mass will be at least 30 percent less than it was when you were thirty-five years old. Without exercise, you'll lose about 1 percent of your muscle mass each year after the age of forty years. To build muscle, don't forget to eat some protein after you have exercised; for example, you could consume 3 oz of meat, drink two cups of skim milk or eat 1 oz of cheese with half cup of beans. Remember that if you have heart disease, diabetes, or high blood pressure, see a doctor (preferably a cardiologist) before you begin any exercise program

Stress Test

A stress test is an electrocardiogram (EKG) that is obtained while you are walking on a treadmill, the speed of which can be controlled. The results of a stress test will tell you how much you can exercise and the strenuousness of the exercise that you can safely perform. Changes will occur during your EKG as the test progresses, and your body responds to the demands of increased exercise. As the monitored level of exercise becomes more strenuous, your heart will require more oxygen and food. If your heart vessels dilate so that blood flow increases, then you can continue with the stress test. However, a blocked or narrowed blood vessel or a spasm of the heart vessels will be revealed in the results of your EKG, and you may experience symptoms of those conditions during the test.

During a stress test, the symptoms of a low blood supply to the heart include the following:

- Headache
- Feeling faint
- Dizziness
- Pain in the left side of your chest or neck or in your left arm
- Pain in the middle of your upper back
- Cold sweats
- A feeling that you are unwell

If you experience any of those symptoms, you must immediately stop your stress test.

Do not exercise if you are in any of the conditions below:

- After a heart attack until you have obtained your cardiologist's approval
- If you have congestive heart failure until you have obtained your doctor's approval
- If you have asthma and you have just taken an antiasthma medication, you are exposed to substances that trigger your asthma, or you are in a very warm or a very cold area
- If you have recently undergone surgery
- If you have exercise anaphylaxis, which is a rare condition involving low blood pressure caused by exercising

Before you start exercising, you should know your maximum heart rate and when to stop working out.

Use the following formula to determine your maximum pulse rate or heart rate per minute:

Subtract your age in years from 220.

Let's say your age is sixty years, then, 220 - 60 = 160.

If you are healthy, then
160 × 60 percent = 96 beats per minute.

In two weeks, determine how much you can safely increase your pulse rate as follows:
160 × 80 percent = 128 beats per minute.

If you are athletic and young, then add 10 percent to that pulse rate.

If you have a negative health factor, like diabetes or mild to moderate high blood pressure well controlled, then 160 × 60 percent = 96 beats per minute.

If you are fifty years old and you have a disease, then 220 - 50 × 60 percent = 102 beats per minute.

If you are fifty years old and are healthy, then 220 - 50 × 80 percent = 136 beats per minute.

You can check the pulse of your radial artery, which is located on the front of your wrist at the base of your thumb. See the picture below.

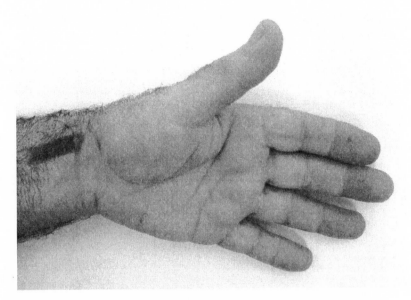

The black line indicates the location of the left radial artery

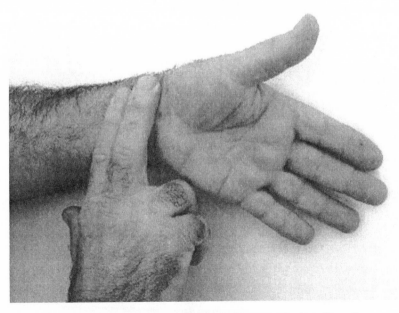

To count your pulse, put the tip of your right hand's index
and middle fingers over the black line area. After you feel the
pulse, count the pulsation of the artery for one minute.

You can also determine your blood pressure and pulse rate with a portable electric automatic device called a sphygmomanometer, and you can check your oxygen and pulse with a small finger-type pulse oximeter. During your daily exercise session, you should check your pulse rate every five minutes when you start. If your blood pressure value is higher than usual, it is okay because blood pressure usually increases during exercise. Be worried, however, if your blood pressure decreases during exercise. A systolic blood pressure value of less than 90 is serious. Check your blood pressure again, and if it is still low, call for help. Some young people less than twenty-five and sometimes the lucky sixty-year-olds have a blood pressure around 92 to 95. In those people, systolic blood pressure value in the low ninety is common during exercise.

Here is another test for those who are older than forty years, healthy, and physically inactive:

Check your pulse rate (let's say that it is eighty), and then exercise.

Your maximum pulse should be calculated as follows:
220 - your age in years × 60 percent

If you are forty years old, then
220 - 40 × 60 percent = 108 beats per minute

After five minutes, stop exercising and check your pulse rate. If it is still lower than 108, exercise more till you reach a pulse of 108.

Stop exercising for six minutes and check your pulse rate again. If it is eighty beats or fewer per minute, then you are okay and you can resume exercising. Begin at a slow and steady pace until you can exercise in fifteen-minute sessions three times weekly. This will improve your muscle function and balance. Over one month, increase the strenuousness of your routine so that you reach 80 percent of your maximum pulse rate. At that point, you will have completed the muscle-toning phase of your program and can advance to the cardiovascular exercise phase.

During your first cardiovascular exercise session, calculate your pulse rate as follows:

> 220 - your age in years (e.g., 40) × 80 percent = 144 beats per minute

If your pulse decreases to a rate within the normal range in fewer than six minutes, then you are physically fit, and you can increase your level of exercise. If your pulse returns to the normal range in eight to ten minutes, then you are moderately physically fit, and you should begin your exercise program slowly and advance it slowly. If your pulse returns to the normal range in more than ten to twelve minutes, see a cardiologist.

Here are some general facts to remember about exercising:

- Obtain medical clearance from your doctor before you work out.
- Walk thirty minutes per day, three to five days a week.
- Jog (for the healthy and medically cleared) fifteen minutes per day, three to five times a week.
- A systolic blood pressure value of less than 90 is serious.
- In young people, a blood pressure of 90 is common and is usually not a sign of ill health.

Walking

- At first, walk fifteen minutes per day.
- Walking for ninety minutes confers the benefits of running for thirty minutes.
- Increase your walking distance by 10 percent per week.
- Walking is less injurious and less stressful for knee joints than is running.
- Walk on grass or clean sidewalks.
- Check your pulse rate every ten minutes while you are walking for the first few days of walking.
- Stop walking if you become short of breath or dizzy or if you experience chest pain, even if you are sure that your discomfort is a stomachache or gastric reflux. Get a checkup. If you can't talk, it means to stop now and sit.

Running

Be careful when running if you are overweight or with any chronic disease. If you have poor vision, don't run in an unfamiliar area.

Running

- improves muscles tone and bulk,
- decreases stress, and
- is inexpensive.

When compared with a forty-year-old who engages in no physical activity, a marathon runner has greater muscle bulk and is stronger. Exercising at a young age will help to maintain your muscle mass when you are older. It is very important to exercise your thigh muscles because they help you to move, they protect you from injury if you fall, and they help you to run if you are in danger. Do you remember when we said that beans are the meat of the poor? Running is the exercise of the poor.

Swimming

- Although it can be difficult for many people to enjoy the luxury of swimming, that form of exercise is often available in America.
- Swimming is a low-impact exercise, but it can be performed vigorously.
- It is healthful for those with arthritis and joint disease because water supports the swimmer's body.
- It can increase flexibility, muscle bulk, and tone; and its effects enhance physical appearance.
- Swimming two to three times per week, which enables your muscles to recover from each session, is beneficial for most people who are not professional or competitive swimmers.

Skating

- Skating is like running and aerobic exercises; it is high impact but with more injuries.
- Skating is a cold, strenuous sport that is good for young people.
- During skating sessions, don't exceed more than 60 percent of your maximum pulse rate if you are not a regular skater.

Dancing

- Dancing is mildly aerobic.
- Work on the pace of your dancing. Again if you can't talk, it means you have to sit down and rest. (Could you please provide more information about this statement?)
- Sit down if you begin to perspire unusually heavily or you experience shortness of breath.

Biking

- Biking is like running for thigh and leg muscle strengthening, but it is less stressful for the joints.
- It develops the thigh muscles.
- Biking slowly and for longer periods is most beneficial.
- Biking too fast reduces its muscle-toning effect.
- If you are healthy, engage in biking on a moderately frequent basis.

Aerobic Exercise and Jumping

- If you are older than fifty years, obtain your doctor's okay before you begin an aerobic exercise program and exercise under the supervision of a trainer rather than alone.
- Know your maximum pulse rate and how to check it.
- Know when to stop a session that involves aerobic and/or jumping exercises.
- If you have been physically inactive, perform aerobic exercises and jumping only four to five minutes a day for three to five days a week, and then increase those exercise periods by three to five minutes weekly.

- Exercising aerobically and jumping for fifteen to thirty minutes three times per week is good for most healthy people.

Weights

Start by lifting small weights. Increase the weight that you lift by one pound per week.

Stretching

Stretching is a popular exercise for people older than forty years regardless of whether they have a disease or a medical condition. Stretching does not increase muscle mass, but it increases and improves joint mobility and flexibility.

The Farmer's Son's Exercises

To farmers, exercise comes naturally.
They walk uphill
And walk downhill.
They walk a few miles every day.
They push and pull.
They plant trees
And cut trees.
To plow the land, they use a mule or a bull.
They cut the fruits
And go to town to sell them.
They really work. All of them work.
The kids, the mom, the dad.

The daughters cook
And serve the lunch
To those who work
The working force.
Life is a choice,
And I love this choice.

Not everyone can have a farm
Or learn to farm.
Here in the USA we have cars;
Everyone has a car.
Our work on Wall Street
Or in hospitals
Or on computers takes a lot of time.
If we do not exercise, we can say an early farewell
To those who love us.

So how can we have the benefits of a healthy farmer's life? When you are older than forty years and have no time for training in clubs, you can follow the farmer's son's exercises to have a healthy life.

Just let me remind you, simply put, there are three types of exercises:

1. Toning, stretching, and flexibility exercise
2. Strenuous aerobic cardiovascular exercise
3. Weight lifting to increase muscle bulk

The farmer's son's exercises are a combination of these three types of exercise.

Toning and stretching are simple, and they are beneficial exercises if you'd like to have a shapely body and your weight under control. Toning and stretching are also good for people with certain physical limitations because those exercises can be modified to accommodate various conditions.

Strenuous cardiovascular exercise is physically challenging, and you should know your physical limitations before you start. If you are older than forty years, you should also know where to go and whom to call if an emergency occurs while you are exercising.

The farmer's son's exercises are a combination of toning, stretching, muscle strengthening, and moderate cardiovascular exercise. They can benefit those of us who are older than forty years and have no time to exercise but who want to live long and stay healthy. They are also inexpensive to perform, and you can do them at home.

To perform the farmer's son's exercises, you need the following weights:

- A 1 lb ring for toning
- A 2.5 to 5 lb covered dumbbell (uncovered metal is cold and unpleasant to touch)
- A roll of plastic for back exercises

And have a different size—small and large—softballs for hand exercise. Buy an electric blood pressure machine to check your blood pressure and pulse before and every five minutes after you start the exercise to make you familiar with your maximum pulse and the increase of your blood pressure.

You begin these exercises by toning all your muscles. Ten to fifteen minutes three times a week without weights, do stretching, deep breathing, body twisting while standing, and mimic boxing (for five minutes). Then begin to perform a mild aerobic exercise while carrying the dumbbells—small, 2.5 to 5 lb for men and the 1 lb ring for women—for five minutes. First, hold the 1 lb weight in each hand; work on the wrist, shoulders, upper back, lower back, hips and legs (see the DVD); and follow that routine for four weeks. During your first exercise session, note your maximum pulse rate and your exercise time limits. Next, increase the weight that you hold in each hand while exercising to 2.5 lb and then, after three weeks, if your condition permits, increase to 5 lb or you can stay on with 2.5 lb. If you are older than sixty years, maintain that routine indefinitely as long as you feel you can do it. If you are younger than fifty years and are strong, hold four to five pounds in each hand while you perform the aerobic exercises. Note your maximum pulse rate and follow your instinct. If you get tired, you are breathing fast, and you can't talk while exercising, stop and rest, check pulse, then next time, reduce the weights or the time you exercise. In few sessions you will know your capacity, and remember, don't overdo it; we want you to be healthy and not to be a wrestler.

It will be available on DVD
I will try to describe the exercises, but as they say, a picture is better than one thousand words.

While standing in the family room with cotton socks on and without the shoes, wearing a short or long pants is no problem, feel comfortable, watch TV (carpeted floors are better to avoid falls), start slow then increase the exercise time. No high jumping to avoid high-impact knee injury. Doing exercise five days a week, eight minutes a day is okay. No need for seven days a week, and no need for thirty minutes a day. In fact, if you exercise five minutes few times a day, it is more beneficial. In three weeks, start moving forward and backward and sideways to improve your muscles strength, reflexes, balance, and bone strength—to survive in case you fall. Balance depends on a functioning vision, feet sensations, strong reflexes, internal ear sensetivity, and the functioning CEO, the brain, since getting older has its problems. Your reflexes get slower 1 percent per bulk your muscles lose, 1 percent per year, and brain diseases start slowly like parkinsonism and Alzheimer's. Exercise can improve muscle bulk, reflex time, balance; and all these can improve the brain in its CEO decisions to keep you out of accidents.

You can perform the farmer's son's exercises during a fast walk or walking with a backpack uphill and downhill. You have to have good vision and have to be familiar with the area to avoid accidents. Again, home exercise is better; and you might move forward, backward, and side to side while carrying weights.

Push-ups

If you are older than twenty years and you are healthy, then push-ups are a good addition to your exercise routine. If you are over fifty, do push-ups as in the DVD while standing against the wall or a well-fixed kitchen table or in the shower under warm water (free hot packs).

Achilles Tendon Stretch

Do it on the wall or in the shower. See the DVD.
Have your feet well fixed on the ground so that you do not slip.

In the shower, say you have pain in between shoulders, let the warm water hit the area while your hands are pushing the wall and moving as standing push-ups. Give it few minutes, not seconds; it is like hot packs, except your muscles are moving. To stretch your calf muscles, see the position again. While holding the wall with both hands, move leg, the right leg, backward. Touching the ground, the left foot will be touching the wall and stretch the right leg by moving the body forward and backward, then switch legs. See DVD exercise.

This exercise stretches the Achilles tendon, making your ankle more flexible. Keep the warm water hitting your calf muscles—it improves leg circulation.

If you have peripheral neuritis without poor circulation, let the warm water hit your legs—front and back—and feet. The warm water dilates the small vessels and brings more blood to the feet, which is the farthest part of the body from the heart, and are therefore prone to poor circulation.

You can supplement the exercise plan described above by walking in your neighborhood for fifteen minutes each day. After a few weeks of following that plan, you can increase your walking pace. Whether you live in the suburbs or in the city, be sure to walk at times and in places that are likely to be safe.

Avoiding Exercise-Related Complications

- Warm up first.
- Remember that several brief periods of mild exercise are more productive than a brief, strenuous, high-impact exercise session.
- Weight lifting is okay, but exercises that develop mobility are best for people with physical limitations. If you have a

disorder or disease, be sure to obtain your doctor's approval before you begin weight lifting.

- Take supplementary antioxidants and omega-3 fatty acids and drink water. Sodium and potassium are needed if it is hot or if you are sweating a lot. Take half banana or a half cup of orange juice for the potassium and four pretzels for the sodium.

Exercise and Health Conditions

If you have any of the following disorders, conditions, or diseases, you must obtain your doctor's approval before you begin any exercise program:

- Diabetes
- Heart disease
- Peripheral vascular disease
- Obesity
- Hypertension
- Long-term smoking
- A recent fracture
- Arthritis
- Parkinson's disease
- Chronic fatigue syndrome
- Deep venous thromboses (Clots in the leg's deep veins; it is a disaster if not treated.)
- Asthma
- Pregnancy
- Recent surgery
- Incipient surgery
- Pulmonary disease
- Recent childbirth

Remember that if you have a health problem like one of those listed above, you should not perform any strenuous exercise; it could kill you instead of helping you. Strenuous exercise is not for you. Exercise that is too rigorous can increase the levels of free radicals and the risk for blood clotting. It can also cause dizziness and/or muscle pain. High-impact aerobic exercise can worsen the effects of degenerative diseases and may cause injury. Urinary incontinence can develop in women who exercise too strenuously. For those individuals, exercises that have a mild-to-moderate impact are best. Also remember that age can be a negative factor with respect to exercise, so don't overdo it!

I want you to exercise throughout the day few minutes at a time while you're in the shower, cooking, or watching TV. You can exercise five to eight minutes at a time before a meal or one hour after a meal and three hours before you sleep as well as when you awake in the morning. Watch for opportunities to exercise throughout the day. Just keep this in mind: if you want to live a longer and healthier life, exercise!

Type 2 Diabetes and Exercise

During exercise in diabetics, the pulse goes up (know your maximum pulse). Also, the blood pressure goes up (stops at 160/100) and blood sugar goes down. Keep blood sugar above 120, very low sugar (below 60) is dangerous. Do not trust your machine when it says 80; it may be in fact lower (finger prick sugar is higher than blood drawn from the elbow area 8 to 12 percent).

Diabetics who are athletes, you can deplete the stored glycogen in the liver in one hour; and to restore it, you need 500 calories of carbohydrate. And it takes twenty-four hours to restore this amount as glycogen in the liver, that's why we suggest exercising every other day. And since carbohydrates are the main foods for energy, to avoid low sugar, take 100-calorie carbohydrate one to two hours before you exercise and keep juice, Gatorade, or sweets with you all times including in the car while going back to your home to avoid accidents from low sugar.

If you have type 2 diabetes, you must take some precautions before you exercise. First, your doctor must evaluate you to determine your maximum pulse rate, and he or she may refer you to a nutritionist for dietary advice. After you have received your medical clearance to exercise, you can walk before or after meals. For example, you could exercise for five to ten minutes several times a day one to two hours after a meal. You may lose weight, and you might require less or no drug therapy. For those of us with diabetes, exercise is the cheapest and best medicine. However, remember that if you have diabetes and your HbA1c value (which reflects your blood sugar level over the two prior months) is higher than eight, do not exercise until that value is seven or lower.

Remember that exercise increases insulin sensitivity and uses blood sugar for energy. It will reduce the blood sugar, especially if you just took insulin-stimulant medications like Glucotrol and you did not eat or ate a little.

Those who are strong and young who exercise for an hour, avoid developing low blood sugar level. Check blood sugar before exercise. If it is around 100, take 100 calories of high-glycemic-index carbohydrates and exercise after one hour. Check your sugar every thirty minutes if you want to exercise more than one hour (the young and well-controlled diabetes). Others suggest sugar pills, candy, or soft drinks. The farmer's son suggests this:

1. Take one tablespoon of honey (60 calories) with a two thumb-size whole grain bread (30 calories). Honey is stored in your muscles and will be used when you start the exercise.
2. Or take the sterile at any time, a small-size banana (80 calories). The advantage of banana soothes the stomach. No bloating, no need for cleaning. Its glycemic index is higher than sugar (sugar GI is 73 while a ripe banana is 100, equal to glucose pills). It has the highest potassium in all fruits and soft drinks, which you need after sweating.
3. Take four pretzels to cover for the sodium loss.
4. Take one vitamin E or Protegra (vitamins A, E, C, selenium and zinc). It neutralizes your free radicals. If your blood sugar is 140, take half this amount and one pill of vitamins.
5. Those who have muscle pain, on insulin stimulants, or on statins, a 30 mg of CoQ10 is indicated after exercise.

If the blood sugar is 220, take one cup of water and the anti oxidant pill; and in thirty minutes of exercise, check blood sugar. If it is less than 140 and you want to exercise another half hour, take half banana and three pretzels and a cup of water.

Also, the antioxidant vitamins I mentioned are good for those who have no disease, are over forty, and are doing strenuous exercise over one hour.

If you have diabetes, avoiding episodes of low blood sugar (hypoglycemia) is always important. Before you exercise, check your blood sugar level (which should be around 120 if you exercise without having eaten). Remember that the blood sugar value from the vein in your elbow is lower than the value from your finger prick sugar. If your blood sugar level is low, then consume some calories in the form of sugar tablets, eight ounces juice, one tablespoon honey, a ripened banana, or candy if nothing else is available. If you burn sixty more calories during a fifteen-minute workout, you will have used the food value of a half cup of orange juice. Keep sweets in your pocket when you exercise if you have no banana or juice, and remember that the symptoms of low blood sugar can develop quickly and are more dangerous than those produced by a high blood sugar level.

If you have diabetes but you are young and strong, then you can expend over three hundred calories per hour during moderate exercise. In that case, keep some juice and candy handy or take one tablespoonful of honey before exercise. Honey is stored in the muscles; it is used before the fat for energy, reducing the ketones.

Signs of low sugar in the blood are sweating, dizziness, nervousness, irritability, and the most important one is sudden blurry vision and palpitation.

Take a high-glycemic-index carbohydrate. Even before you check your blood sugar, remember nobody dies from high sugar in minutes or hours even if it is five hundred; but low sugar can give accidents and heart arrhythmia, breathing difficulty, and, at a very low sugar (less than 45), seizure and coma. In a short time, it is a blessing for type 2 diabetics on oral medications; they have less incidence for low sugar than insulin-dependent patients. You need 100 calories immediately, equal to a cup of juice or four to eight solid candies. Notice if you have low sugar without exercise, you need half of this amount because you do not have the increased metabolic rate caused by the exercise. Use a tablespoonful of honey. Sixty calories before exercise can reduce the incidence of low sugar.

Remember the following:

- Drink water one to two cups every thirty minutes even if you are not thirsty.
- Don't exercise in hot or cold weather.
- It is suggested to carry a cell phone and wear a necklace with your medical information.
- Don't exercise if you have bleeding retinopathy; it really can make the condition worse. And don't exercise if you are after glaucoma surgery. Don't carry any heavy object. Period.
- Don't exercise after any abdominal, thoracic, bone, or head operation till the doctor approves it.
- You may lose 600 cc of water per hour during a strenuous exercise. Take a cup of water every thirty minutes before you get thirsty.
- Thirst indicate, dehydration or loss of 2 percent of your body water (around 850 cc). In this case, don't replace it with water only; you need sodium, potassium, and water (e.g., Gatorade).
- Also, you need potassium and sodium before or during a moderate exercise or after sweating—four pretzels (each 80 mg salt, 8 mg potassium, and 20 calories) and a half cup of orange juice (240 mg potassium) or medium banana (600 mg potassium).

Avoid Developing a High Blood Sugar Level

If you are diabetic, remember that a high blood sugar level (hyperglycemia) causes insulin deficiency, overeating, and failure to take prescribed medications.

If your blood sugar level is higher than 200, wait before you exercise if you have just eaten or take your medications as prescribed.

Heart Disease and Exercise

Because diabetes, high blood pressure, and high levels of bad cholesterol affect the heart negatively and because exercise can protect against the effects of those conditions, then exercising is likely to decrease the risk of cardiovascular diseases. Exercise improves the function of your heart, which becomes stronger, and it lowers your pulse rate because your body receives more oxygen and nutrition with less work from your heart. As a result, you will feel better and work better.

If you have heart disease (regardless of whether you have diabetes), then you must be careful before, during, and after exercising; and you may need advice about exercise management from your doctor, a physiotherapist, or a nutritionist. The American Heart Association suggests that a low-fat diet and exercise are part of a healthful lifestyle. Remember that exercise is a cost-effective way to increase your level of good cholesterol, especially if you are overweight and should lose a few pounds. You can exercise with dumbbells while lying down with your head on a pillow. The more rigorous the exercise, the better (in general); but any exercise is better than no exercise. Let me tell you why.

Many of us tend not to exercise when we are under stress, but waiting until we feel mentally ready to exercise can be a mistake. Exercise relieves emotional stress and even improves sleep. If we exercise when we are facing challenges and uncertainty, we will help ourselves to remain mentally and physically fit and to better manage adversity. We will also set an excellent example for family members and friends.

Obesity and Exercise

Just remember one thing: exercise alone can strengthen muscles, can reduce stress, and can improve circulation but may not have too much effect on weight. And remember that walking around the pyramids in Egypt, the calories spent were neutralized with a cup of sugarcane juice (a tasty sweet from sugarcane's juice is high in sugar), but exercise plus a diet plan with less calories will decrease weight more than the diet alone. Obese people are in a continuous exercise; it is their extra weight. A person who weighs 120 lb spends 140 calories if he walks slowly for an hour, but a 200 lb person will spend 200 calories.

Exercise among the obese depends on the age to avoid knee injuries; swimming, strengthening exercises with small weights while sitting, walking, and the best is the farmer's type exercise—gardening, digging, racking leaves, planting roses, and grass mowing (avoid snow shoveling).

If you have no land around your house, do push-ups while standing against a wall in the house or in the shower to mimic the racking and digging. Have two dumbbells, 2.5 lb each, bend a little forward, and move it side to side, up and down. Please see the DVD.

People who are preparing to undergo weight loss (bariatric) surgery are often advised to perform some degree of regular exercise, even if it involves only walking for fifteen minutes and then increasing the number of those brief exercise sessions each day. Having a trainer is even better. Following an exercise program before surgery can enhance postsurgical results. When compared with their physically fit counterparts, unfit patients often spend more days in the hospital and may experience more complications such as a DVT. Those blood clots are among the most preventable and deadly complications that can develop after bariatric surgery or in immobile patients, and they are more likely to occur in the pelvic veins than in the veins of the legs. Appropriate postsurgical mobility and activity definitely reduce the risk for DVT. In addition, cardiac myopathy may develop in some patients (particularly those who are obese), and arrhythmia and/or low cardiac output can occur. Exercise (as directed by a doctor) protects against the development of those conditions too. It can also increase metabolism and reduce the likelihood of excessive blood clotting.

Asthma and Exercise

In America today, ten million Americans have chronic or seasonal asthma. If you have that common disorder, remember the following:

- A well-controlled asthmatic, with no recent attacks, can exercise like healthy people; asthmatics usually live longer than diabetics.

- Do not exercise if you have even a questionable asthma attack.
- Avoid exercising in cold weather because cold narrows the bronchi (air passages) in the lungs.

Alcoholism and Exercise

In people who are addicted to alcohol (as in those who are not), exercise (walking, yoga) has the following effects:

- Decreases anxiety
- Improves brain function
- Improves muscle tone
- Sets a positive example of a healthful lifestyle

Exercise that is directed by a physiotherapist may be best for people with alcoholism.

Parkinson's disease and Exercise

This is usually under supervision to avoid falls. In people with Parkinson's disease, exercise, improves flexibility, improves muscle tone, improves joint mobility, strengthens muscles, and thus protects against fractures.

If you have Parkinson's disease, remember to

- carry a cane to help maintain balance;
- walk in a familiar area;
- avoid bumps and holes;
- consider walking, stretching, and/or exercising under the guidance of a physiotherapist.

Pregnancy and Exercise

For most women, exercising before and after pregnancy is beneficial, depending on the trimester (early or late). Some facilities or health clubs have special programs for pregnant women in which exercise decreases constipation, improves flexibility and joint movement, reduces stress, and improves the quality of sleep.

If you are pregnant, be sure to call your doctor before you begin to exercise if you have high blood pressure, vaginal bleeding, or a history of premature delivery.

Preferable forms of exercise for pregnant women include the following and to exercise in groups under supervision.

- Walking
- Swimming
- Stretching

If you are pregnant, remember the following:

- Start exercising slowly and as your doctor directs.
- Increase your exercise slowly each week as directed by your doctor.
- Avoid jumping and bouncing.
- Stop if you feel dizzy or tired or if palpitations develop.

Arthritis and Exercise

If you have knee arthritis, exercise can be beneficial, but you must avoid causing joint friction and placing pressure on your knees. Before you exercise, take an anti-inflammatory medication. In addition, taking a supplement containing glucosamine and chondroitin can be helpful. Swimming, which is a no weight-bearing exercise, is good for people with arthritis because it does not adversely affect the joints. Some floor exercises that you can perform while you are lying on your back on a soft floor cover may also be of benefit. If you have arthritis, avoid jogging or jumping (and playing volleyball).

Swimming is good for arthritis; it is a nonweight-bearing exercise and all leg and thigh muscles are used (flexors, extensors, and the butt muscles).

If you have knee pain caused by osteoarthritis, a cane can help; energy-absorbing shoes, elastic bandage, brace or knee sleeve can help to stabilize the knee

Do nonweight-bearing exercises while lying flat such as water exercises, hot packs, or electric heat pads, then do stretching as well as range of motion and flexibility exercises.

Be sure you don't have a meniscus tear, which is the weight-absorbing cartilage located between the thigh and leg bones.

Treatment by all meds is ineffective except for short period.

Glucosamine and chondroitIn—OTC—help in the early stages.

Take no steroidal anti-inflammatory drugs Motrin, Alieve, and Advil thirty minutes before exercise.

Cortisone injections by a doctor and the better, cheaper hyaluronic acid injections in the knee have good results.

Sit on a chair and do strengthening exercises to the upper body. Move the foot and toes in flexion and extension movements while sitting on the chair. Move the knee slowly if you have no pain and see an orthopedic doctor.

Chronic Fatigue Syndrome and Exercise

Chronic fatigue syndrome is associated with brain function rather than muscle function. People with that disorder can exercise on the days on which they have less pain. Physiotherapy is a good option as are treatments with ultrasound (which provide deep heat), hot soaks (which provide superficial heat), nerve stimulation (which improves muscle tone), and bandaging (which supports painful joints and muscles and facilitates movement). Physiotherapy can also relieve insomnia and improve sleep in people with chronic fatigue syndrome, and taking the supplement coenzyme Q10 (CoQ10) 50 to 100 mg before exercise, which is usually low in the muscles when having this disease. It is the spark for the mitochondria (the energy factory for each cell) to produce energy and improve muscle pain.

Fractures and Exercise

Your doctor may prescribe exercises that can help you recover from a fracture, but be sure to proceed only according to his or her orders. You may have to be seen by a physiatrist. Remember one thing: fracture of the spine, hip, and femur kills by giving blood clots in the calf, thigh, or pelvic veins; and the reason is immobility. A blood thinner usually is prescribed; take it on time and follow up with your doctor.

Hypertension and Exercise

If you have hypertension, don't consume caffeine or eat salty foods such as pickles, salty soups, pretzels, or salty peanuts before you exercise. You want to keep your levels of potassium and calcium high and your level of sodium low. Do not exercise if your systolic blood pressure value is higher than 160 or your diastolic blood pressure is higher than 95. Your blood pressure will increase further during exercise, and that will stress your heart and may cause a coronary spasm. Do not shovel snow, jog, or (if you are elderly) walk too fast, especially if it is cold. When the weather is bad, exercise at home and let the younger family members shovel the snow from sidewalks and driveways. If you sweat a lot during exercise, you can consume some sports drinks containing salt, and don't forget that sodium is found naturally in many foods (even orange juice, which contains about 30 mg per 8 oz serving). If you perspire excessively during exercise, stop and eat four pretzels in addition to a cup of water every fifteen minutes.

Rules for All People Who Want to Exercise

- To avoid dehydration, drink one cup of water every fifteen to twenty minutes while exercising. If you are young and strong, exercising for one or two hours, drink a cup of juice or an 8 oz. sports drink, which contains sodium in it in addition to water.
- Avoid exercising in low temperatures or high temperatures and don't exercise if you have a fever.
- If you are walking, be sure that you know how to return to your point of departure and walk with a friend if possible.
- Regardless of whether you have diabetes, carry some water, some candy and a cell phone.
- Resistance exercises are good for the elderly and those with certain health problems such as inabilities.

CHAPTER 3

A Checklist of Healthful Food
Milk, Cheese, Meat, Beans,
Oil and Whole Grains

In this chapter, we'll continue our review of familiar foods and beverages as well as exotic herbs and spices that add nutrition and flavor to a healthful diet.

Percentage daily value written on a food label is defined as the recommended daily allowance (RDA) of a certain food component to help the consumer plan a healthy diet.

The percent daily value of a nutrient written on a label is the content of a certain essential macronutrients—protein, carbohydrate, and fat or micronutrients like calcium, vitamins (A and C), and sodium present in a serving of a certain food. This percentage is calculated for a person who needs 2,000 calories a day.

To know how many calories you need at rest, multiply your weight in pounds by 10.

So if you are 100 pounds, you need 1,000 calories, and your DV should be half what is written on the labels percent DV unless you want to increase your weight.

If you are 200 pounds and inactive, you need 2,000 calories per day.

If you are 200 lb and doing a heavy construction work eight hours per day, you may need 3,500 to 4,000 calories per day, and your percentage should be doubled.

If you are active, add calories according to the type of work or intensity per hour. Running is 600 calories while walking fast is 200 calories per hour (80 calories for sedentary life).

- Which Food Is Better for You to Eat?

High-calorie or low-calorie food? Which fats—high-protein or low-protein foods?

First, let us start with our body's minimal needs per day. We will start with the recommended DVA (daily value allowance for energy-producing nutrients) in grams for a person who needs 2,000 calories per day.

- Total fat is less than 65 grams (saturated fat, less than 20 grams). Each gram of fat gives 9 calories; it's around 600 calories or 30 percent calories of daily allowance.
- Total carbohydrate is 300 g. Each gram gives 4 calories; therefore 1,200 calories or 60 percent of total calories.
- Total protein of 50 g. Each gram is 4 calories totals to 200 calories or 10 percent of daily calories.

Daily value of fiber is over 25 grams per day.

Percent DV for minerals, vitamins, and trace elements are in grams, milligrams, and micrograms. These compounds are usually over-the-counter. It will give you an idea how much you need per day if you are healthy, no disease, and not deficient in any of these nutrients, minerals, vitamins, and micronutrients daily value.

- Cholesterol less than 300 mg per day
- Sodium less than 2,400 mg
- Potassium 3,500 mg
- Calcium 1,000 to 1,200 mg
- Phosphorus 1,000 mg
- Magnesium 400 mg
- Zinc 15 mg
- Iron 18 mg
- Copper 2 mg
- Manganese 2 mg
- Chromium 120 mcg
- Selenium 70 mcg
- Iodine 150 mcg

Percent Daily Value of Vitamins

- 5,000 IU vitamin A
- 60 mg vitamin C (You can take 100 times of this amount if indicated.)
- 400 IU vitamin D (More than 1,000 IU may give toxicity in few weeks.)
- 30 IU vitamin E (maximum 1,000 IU, if per day)
- 80 mcg vitamin K
- 20 mg niacin (as medicine up to 2 g per day)
- 2 mg vitamin B6, (up to 100 mg)
- 1.5 mg vitamin B1 (avoid more than 100 mg per day)
- 6 mcg vitamin B12 (can be given intramuscularly 100 mcg in deficiency cases)
- 300 mcg biotin

Serving size means a food content of 80 to 120 calories per cup (e.g., one medium apple, 8 oz cup of juice) or as tablespoonful, teaspoonful, slice, etc.

I will discuss some important foods, proteins, carbohydrates, fats, seeds, fruits, vegetables, spices, and vitamins and minerals.

I will talk about individual foods which you know. I just want to make you aware of what to avoid and how much to eat at a time or a day in case you have a disease before forty or no disease but over forty (and remember life starts after sixty).

Milk

A cup of whole milk contains

88 percent water,
5 percent sugar lactose,
3.5 percent protein, and
3.5 percent fat.

Milk contains minerals like calcium and phosphate and vitamins which fortify milk like vitamin D (400 IU per quart) and vitamin A (2,000 IU per quart). Vitamin A is lost if milk is exposed to the sun or in skim milk because of lack of protection by fat.

Milk and Fat Contents

Skim milk has no fat.
Low-fat milk is 1 percent fat.
Reduced fat has 2 percent fat.
Whole milk is more than 3.5 percent fats.
(Avoid but this is good for people under four years.)

Reduced fat 2 percent milk.

Cows, goats, sheep, and buffaloes produce milk, which is usually found on the breakfast table and anytime during the day. A cup of milk contains (a 244 grams milk is one serving size or 122 calories.)

Saturated fat, 3 g, 10 percent DV, acceptable

Unsaturated fat, 1.3 g, acceptable

Lactose, 95 percent of the total carbohydrate

285 mg calcium, 25 percent DV

105 IU vitamin D, 25 percent DV

Vitamin B2, 25 percent DV

Vitamin B12, 18 percent DV

100 mg sodium, 5 percent DV

460 IU vitamin A. (This vitamin is added to milk.)

one whole milk cup has 3.3 percent fat contents.

With the same nutrition as low fat milk except

Total fat of 8 g (high)

Saturated of 4.5 g. (high) It is 20 percent (not recommended).

Skim milk is better.

A cup has

2 g monounsaturated and 1.5 g polyunsaturated or 8 percent DV, acceptable

Milk can be made into cheese, which is a very nutritious food that is high in calcium (and often high in fat). It's important to remember that soft, raw-milk cheeses can be the source of *salmonella* infection and tuberculosis.

Remember that 8 oz of milk yields 1 oz of cheese (which contains 7 g of protein and 150 to 200 mg of calcium). Skim milk cheese contains 2 percent fat. Pasteurized skim milk cheese is fat free. Milk is a good source of minerals such as calcium and magnesium. Consuming enough calcium every day helps to prevent osteoporosis. Magnesium is effective in reducing the incidence of type 2 diabetes because it increases the ability of insulin to direct sugar metabolism. Some infants younger than one year old are allergic to milk and must drink soy milk. Milk intolerance is common in Mediterranean countries.

Milk contains lactose, a sugar that is digested by the enzyme lactase. People who are deficient in lactase cannot digest lactose, and this causes gas and bloating. Some investigators believe that the high calcium content of milk may reduce the incidence of cancer.

Cheese

Cheese is a calcium and protein factor, but it is the highest source of saturated fat in USA.

Cheese is a solid food made from milk. It is a form of milk minus water and minus sugar (water is 88 percent of milk, and sugar is 3.5 percent) made by adding acidic vinegar or lemon juice. This will give the milk curd or coagulum.

Most of cheeses are made by the less acidic culture bacteria, which feeds on sugar, giving the lactic acid. When you add acid to milk, it gives a curd (coagulum). They add the enzyme rennet with heat and mechanical stirring of the coagulated curd. Then the curd is compressed to give the solid cheese we eat. Cheese can be soft, fresh with short shelf life or semisoft, hard, and extra hard with a longer shelf life. It can be colored, flavored, or spiced with garlic and lemon. It can be called by the source of milk like goat or sheep cheese.

The most common cheese eaten in the USA is the processed cheese, the one in which salt, calcium, and preservatives were added to it.

What is important to know about cheese is that Americans doubled their cheese intake from 14 lb in 1970 to 28 lb in 2000, but the Greek and French ate more than 45 lb per year. If eating more fat gives more heart attacks, how come we have the French paradox we mentioned? They have fewer cardiovascular diseases than the USA. The reason is the black grapes and red wine content of resveratrol, which dilates the coronaries, plus they eat less calories per meal (25 percent less calories), that's why only 5 percent of the French are obese. They also eat olive oil and more beans in their diet.

Cheese Label: What Is Important to Know When You Read It?

You have to check the label for calcium content—the higher the better.

Avoid sodium content (salty cheese) if you have high blood pressure. Cheese has low or no sugar lactose since bacteria used it, giving lactic acid during the process of making the cheese. Cheddar cheese has 5 percent of the lactose while aged cheese has none. So for diabetics, low-fat cheese has high protein, reasonable amount of fat, and no carbohydrate. Protein and fat do not need insulin to be metabolized.

Each 8 oz (one cup) of milk gives 1 oz cheese. The difference is the amount of sugar and calorie content. In a cup of milk, there is 12 g sugar lactose while 1 oz of cheese made from the same milk has less than 3 g of sugar.

Some cheeses may have 14 g of fat in 1.5 oz with 9 g saturated fat.

So read the label and know what you want.

For diabetic, overweight, and hypertensive patients, low-fat cheese is better than milk since it has lower calories and minimal sugar.

Low-salt cheese means 32 mg sodium in 4 oz or 0.25 percent DV.

For high cholesterol, eat low-fat cheese or skim milk.

For osteoporosis, eat low-fat cheeses, skim milk, or soy milk fortified with calcium.

For lactose intolerance (Mediterranean people), hard low-fat cheese is good; it has no lactose, and soft cheese has a small amount of lactose.

What Does Low-fat and Low-sodium Cheese Mean?

Low fat means less than 3 g of fat per serving or 4 oz.

No fat means less than 0.5 g of fat per serving.

Cheeses (less than 2 g fat per 1.5 oz) like cottage cheese, which also has the highest calcium in all cheeses, 370 mg in 1.5 oz, may be better since it has more vitamin A and calcium.

Eat only 3 oz whole milk cheese per week to avoid too much saturated fat, but eat two to three servings of skim milk per day (a serving is one cup of milk) or cheese (1.5 oz each serving).

Cheeses prevent dental caries since it has less or no sugar and may have antibacterial effect.

Soy Milk

Although it is called milk, soy milk is not a dairy product. Some researchers believe that female infants who drink soy milk experience early puberty although that association has not been proven. Here are some facts about soy milk, which is a nutritious beverage that may decrease the incidence of heart disease:

- Its taste is different from that of milk.
- A cup of soy milk, which is calcium fortified, has the same contents of a regular milk, except the advantage of customizing the flavor. Vanilla is good.
- It contains the good fat instead of the saturated fat found in whole milk. It has omega-3 fat.

    1. To vegetarians' advantage, it is a source of protein.
    2. It is less expensive
    3. It reduces menopausal symptoms and has high phytoestrogen contents with anticancer effect
    4. It has fiber of 0.5 g per cup.
    5. It can be fortified with calcium.
    6. It reduces breast and prostate cancer incidence.

- It is a good source of protein.

Serving size :one 8 oz cup

Compare a cup of milk to unsweetened soy milk:

Milk has 120 cal, 5 g total fat, 4 g saturated fat, 125 mg sodium, 8 g protein, 11 g sugar, vitamins A and D, and calcium.

Soy milk has 90 cal, 4 g fat, 0.5 g saturated fat, 30 mg sodium; it has 0.5 to 2 g fiber and 7 g protein. It has 1 g sugar (you have to use soy milk calcium fortified with calcium and vitamin D).

As you see it has low sodium, low sugar, low saturated fats, and high good fats; it has fiber too since it comes from beans. It lacks the calcium and vitamin D.

Soy Cheese

Cheeses made from curdled soybean milk. Sometimes spices and herbs are added to it like garlic, pepper, and salt. It has vitamins A and D.

It is usually fortified with calcium, 200 to 300 mg per ounce.

Each ounce contains 50 calories (it is low), 7 grams protein, 7 grams fats (minimal saturated fats). It has no cholesterol. It is good for people with milk allergy, especially if they have a bone-thinning disease, lactose intolerance, and hyperlipidemia (high fats in the blood). It is especially good for low-vision people who can't read the labels.

- **Edible Animal Meat, Poultry, and Fish as a Source of Protein**

Everybody knows about meat. It is high in protein, B complex vitamins, minerals, especially chromium, zinc, and iron. Liver meat has the highest vitamins and minerals, but it is high in cholesterol.

There is one thing I want to mention: the type of meat this country used to eat just sixty years ago was grass-fed animals. After the animals started feeding on grains and corn, there was an increase in cardiovascular diseases, cancer, and obesity. The reason may be secondary to high meat intake of meat of nongrass-fed animals and taking less fish with reduction in omega-3 fat.

The difference between grass-fed and the grain-fed animals is the 70 percent reduction in the level of conjugated linolenic acid (CLA). The grass fed has double the amount of CLA, which increases metabolism; increases muscle mass; decreases triglycerides; decreases cancer of colon, pancreas, prostate, and skin; and it decreases cardiovascular atherosclerotic disease.

The best meat—grass fed—has high CLA level. Lamb has 5 mg and goat 3 has mg.

The CLA, which is sold as capsules, is made from safflower. It comes in 750 mg, but it may have less effect on the benefits of CLA we mentioned.

So when you eat meat, eat grass-fed animals' meat. Otherwise, at least select lean meat or better extralean meat.

Grill it, roast it, or bake the meat, and avoid frying.

Eat skinless white breast chicken, grilled, the same with turkey. Eat cold-water fish twice a week.

Get proteins from beans, whole grains, and nuts other days.

Lean meat with a serving size of 3.5 oz contains the following:

- 70 percent water
- 150 calories
- 5 to 21 g protein
- 3 to 15 g fat
- 1 to 5 percent minerals

Very lean meat of 3.5 oz contains these:

- 100 calories
- 21 g protein
- 1 to 3 g fat
- fish (the omega-3 factor)

Saturated Fats

While saturated fats are found in meat, dairy products, and food-containing dairy products like butter and margarine, plant oils has saturated fats too. Coconut and palm oil are beneficial to the body unless taken over 7 percent of calorie daily value (20 grams per day or 180 calorie).

Saturated fats are needed for each cell wall structure, energy, and multiple hormones production; but if taken in high amounts, it will increase the bad cholesterol and decrease the good cholesterol with its harmful effects such as atherosclerosis and increase of cardiovascular diseases.

Butter has lecithin, which is antimicrobial, and it contains some trace elements.

Coconut and palm oil contain lauric acid, which is important for brain function and immunity.

Oils

Olive Oil: The best Life Extender
(When I say olive oil, I mean extra virgin olive oil)

The most important part of Mediterranean diet is the omega-9.

Olive oil is a cornerstone of the healthful Mediterranean diet. In antiquity, the versatile olive yielded its oil for use in foods and cooking as a lubricant in cosmetics and soaps, in religious rituals, and as fuel to provide lamplight. Today, olive oil graces the table as a seasoning for salads, is used in many dishes, and is an essential ingredient in a constellation of ethnically diverse dishes. It is available in various brands (each of which has a characteristic color and flavor) from countries including Italy, Spain, Greece, and France. Olive oil is rich in beneficial fats and is an excellent source of omega-9 fatty acid. There are several types of olive oil.

- Extra virgin olive oil is obtained from the first pressing of olives. Extravirgin olive oil has a superior flavor and is most often consumed uncooked. It contains a host of beneficial nutrients, such as beta-carotene, vitamin E, calcium, iron, polyphenols, monounsaturated fatty acids, and antioxidants.
- Virgin olive oil. This oil results from the second pressing of olives and can be used in cooking or consumed uncooked. Extra virgin olive oil is higher in polyphenols, monounsaturated fats, and omega-9 fatty acids.
- Light olive oil. This olive oil, which has a relatively lighter color and flavor, is finely filtered and has a milder taste. Because it has a higher smoke point than the other types of olive oil, this is often used for cooking, baking, and frying.

All olive oil types has the same calories, but the extra virgin has less than 1 percent acidity or less free oleic acid; it is better digested, and because of its aroma, it is eaten in a lesser amount.

Because the omega-9 fatty acid and polyphenols in olive oil decrease the level of bad cholesterol and increase the level of good cholesterol, consuming only two to three tablespoons (preferably of extravirgin olive oil) daily can reduce the risk for cardiovascular diseases. If you try that pleasant therapy and slightly increase your level of exercise to counteract the effect of those extra calories, your level of good cholesterol will increase in as little as one or two months. Olive oil also benefits those with a gastric ulcer or gastritis because it coats and protects the lining of the stomach. It can decrease the risk for gallstones because it stimulates the flow of bile as well as the secretion of pancreatic enzymes

One tablespoonful of virgin olive oil contains 77 percent as monounsaturated, 11 percent as polyunsaturated, and 10 percent as saturated. Compared to one tablespoon of butter, saturated fat content is 66 percent.

Olive oil action, nutrition, and advantages:

- It can reduce the bad cholesterol.
- It increases the good cholesterol.
- It reduces the triglycerides.

While diabetes does the opposite action on cholesterol, so it is good for diabetics.

Also, it doesn't need insulin when used by cells to give energy, and this cholesterol and the antioxidants' action reduce heart disease.

- In southern Europe, they have low incidence of cardiovascular diseases; they use olive oil as the main source of dietary fats.
- It has vitamin E, carotinoids, and polyphenols as antioxidants (antiaging).
- It is a lubricant for the stomach, reduces constipation, and reduces inflammation of joints.

- Alzheimer's is very rare in the Mediterranean area even in the poor areas probably because they use olive oil daily plus zaatar, black seeds, and corcumin spices.
- The FDA allows labels on olive oil. They claim that olive (virgin) oil reduces the risks of heart disease. They add that the dose is two tablespoonfuls per day and that it is to replace saturated fats (animal fats).
- Weight loss. Olive oil can reduce the visceral fat or belly fat (this is the best olive oil action). It enhances the removal of the visceral fat even without exercise, but to get the best results, you have to reduce the milk and meat's saturated fat intake. I mean, to replace the calories from saturated fats by calories from olive oil because this visceral fat gives high cardiac risk (if you remember the apple-shape person) since it is connected to the liver with multiple veins. I mean it is connected with open roads to the liver, flooding the liver (which manufactures the cholesterol) with fats when asked for by certain hormones. These hormones increase in response to hunger.
- The olive oil has a separate function on weight loss. It gives satiety, which means that if you take two tablespoonfuls at 8:00 PM with tomato slices, low-fat cheese, and a half whole grain slice, when you wake up at 7:00 AM you will not feel that hungry. And when you eat two more tablespoons with two white eggs, zaatar, half slice of bread and yogurt, that will give you low appetite for another eight hours although I don't know how the olive oil works on appetite. But as you know hunger is stimulated by the hormone leptin, olive oil probably inhibits leptin. Remember olive oil is acidic. It may give acid like feeling in the throat if you drink it, so soak a piece of whole grain bread with olive oil, then eat it (or eat it with tomato slices or low-fat cheese).

Eating one of the following in between meals is okay even if you don't feel hungry, with green tea and/or coffee with soy milk and a spoonful of honey.

- Apple or orange
- 4 strawberries
- A pear
- broccoli
- Squash
- Cauliflower
- Red sweet pepper
- 12 peanuts
- 6 almonds
- 4 walnut halves
- Some vitamins

Other Vegetable Oils
Soybean, Sunflower, and Canola Oil

Canola Oil

It is used for frying and is made in Canada (Canada oil = canola). It has no saturated fats. Each tablespoon has 125 calories like the olive oil. It has 13 g fats (60 percent monounsaturated and 33 percent polyunsaturated fat) and has vitamin E (7 percent DV) and vitamin K (21 percent DV).

Canola oil used to come from rapeseed and has erucic acid, which is toxic. Now it is produced with 1 percent erucic acid (less than 2 percent is accepted in USDA). A lot of people do not believe that canola oil is beneficial since nobody knows about the real level of that toxic acid and since other oils are available with a better taste too.

Sunflower Oil

It is becoming famous oil; it has 90 percent mono—and polyunsaturated fats (more in monounsaturated oils like olive oil) and 10 percent saturated fat.

It also has vitamin K, magnesium, zinc, and phytosterols, which reduce cholesterol.

Soybean Oil

All oils have the same calories (120 calorie per one tablespoon).

Soybean oil has a total of 88 percent mono—and polyunsaturated fats (like olive oil). Olive oil is higher in monounsaturated fats while soybean oil is higher in polyunsaturated fats. Also, it has vitamin E and K.

Beans, the high glycemic load factor

Serving size of half cup

It is high in protein, high in complex carbohydrate, and low in sodium.

Beans are the meat of the poor. All varieties of beans (which are an excellent source of complex carbohydrates and protein) can be eaten green or dry, and they are high in fiber. There could be a combination of beans and corn, beans and whole wheat, or beans and brown rice.

It supply most of the essential amino acids. The saponins, phytochemicals, fiber (from lignin), calcium, magnesium, and folate in beans reduce the levels of bad cholesterol in the bloodstream. Soaked beans are less likely to cause flatulence.

Beans alone contain no methionine (an essential amino acid), so they must be combined with corn or a grain such as rice to make a complete protein.

In the Middle East, beans are eaten with bread, in India with rice or wheat, and in South America with corn.

Here are some useful facts about beans:

The fiber-soluble portion of the bean absorbs water and then decreases the flow of food in the intestines. That soluble fiber also lowers the level of bad cholesterol in the bloodstream. The insoluble fiber in beans absorbs the bile acids that are secreted by the liver into the small bowel, reducing cholesterol, and the insoluble fibers give a bulky stool. Both functions decrease the levels of bad cholesterol, relieve constipation, and protect against hemorrhoids. Eating beans decreases the risk of heart disease, a fact demonstrated by many Europeans whose diet is high in nuts, beans, grapes, fruit, and wine. In America, however, we eat more meat, potatoes, white bread, and sweets; and that diet has led to a high incidence of obesity, diabetes, and heart disease. If the latter is your diet, please change the way you eat! Here are some facts to remember about beans.

Red Beans

Red beans contain the highest level of antioxidants of all American foods. They have mostly soluble fiber, they are high in folic acid and antioxidants, and they can lower the levels of bad cholesterol in the bloodstream. Red beans are also high in insoluble fiber, which is good for colon cancer prevention, constipation, and diverticulitis of the colon and reduces the likelihood of developing anal fissures and hemorrhoids.

Pinto Beans

Pinto beans are low in sodium and high in potassium. They contain complex carbohydrates but have a high glycemic load, so eat just one-fourth cup at time unless your calorie needs are high. When eaten in a reasonable amount, pinto beans help to lower high blood pressure, and they are a good source of protein for people with gout.

One-half cup of pinto beans contains 750 mg potassium (25 percent DV); high level of vitamin A; and high levels of magnesium, zinc, and folate.

Kidney Beans

Of all beans, kidney beans are highest in the neurotransmitter tryptophan.

A 100 grams provides 84 calories and has no fat. It has 10 percent protein of the daily value. It has also 10 percent daily value in thiamine and manganese. Kidney beans' proteins are also good for people with gout.

Bean Protein

Bean protein, which is made from a combination of red, black, pinto, and kidney beans, are eaten primarily in the Middle East. Bean protein does not cause an elevated level of uric acid. Thus, it is an excellent source of protein for people with gout in whom eating meat causes joint inflammation and a high level of uric acid in the bloodstream. Bean protein has no fat, but it is high in calories from its complex carbohydrate, so it must be eaten in small portions.

Each 85 g serving of bean, which is the equivalent of a half cup of cooked dried beans, contains the following:

- 22 g of carbohydrates
- 12 g of protein (good amount)
- 116 calories (88 calories from carbohydrate)
- 52 mg calcium (low amount)
- 6.7 g of fiber or 25 percent daily value (high amount)
- 12 percent of the daily value of iron (good amount)
- a high percentage of the daily allowance of beta-carotene, manganese, and folic acid
- a high level of antioxidants, flavonoids
- a high amount of polyphenols

Chickpeas: The Manganese and Magnesium Factor

Chickpeas (garbanzo beans) are eaten pickled or as a paste called hummus.

Roasted fresh chickpeas contain dopamine, which is beneficial to parkinsonism. These patients are deficient in dopamine. Chickpeas contain high levels of manganese, magnesium, and folate, and they are high in calories.

Hummus

Hummus is a healthful food that is made from chickpeas paste. It is eaten as a dip and/or in combination with tahini (sesame paste), garlic, lemon juice, basil, and olive oil. Hummus is often offered with hot red pepper powder in the center of the plate, which is usually garnished with pickles, olives, tomato slices, and/or cucumbers. Hummus has a low glycemic index, but it is high in calories, so eat only one-fourth cup at a time. One tablespoon is 14 grams and has 25 calories.

A cup of hummus, which is 250 g, contains the following:

- It has 415 calories, so unless you are a farmer doing a heavy work eight hours a day, eat hummus as dip. It has 24 g fats, 20 g unsaturated (good fats) or 96 percent of the daily value of manganese (which provides energy for every cell mitochondria).
- It has 44 percent of the daily value of magnesium and phosphate (good for the bones). It has a soluble fiber of 15 g or 60 percent DV, which reduces the levels of bad cholesterol and thus protects against heart and vascular diseases.

A high level of folate or 51 percent DV, which decreases the effect of homocysteine, a well-known independent inflammatory factor in vascular disease.

Magnesium—which is a natural calcium channel blocker and also reduces blood pressure, dilates blood vessels, improves nutrition to the tissues, decreases the levels of the worst type of cholesterol (very low-density lipoprotein—VLDL) and triglyceride—improves insulin sensitivity and works with calcium to build bone.

Each tablespoon is 14 grams and contains 23 calories, so eat two tablespoons at a time if you are not a heavy worker; it is very nutritious.

Fava Beans

Fava beans have the tryptophan factor or the pleasure factor. A 100 g mature edible seeds contain 250 mg tryptophan.

I refer to fava beans as "the levodopa factor." The levodopa in fava beans is a source of the neurotransmitter dopamine, which is also synthesized in the body and is found in the brain.

It is good for Parkinsonism patients. Aging reduces the tryptophan-secreting cells; this gives the fingers and hands repeated involuntary movement at rest.

Because eating a diet that is too high in fava beans can cause obesity, you should eat only a fist-sized amount of them each day. They are good for people who have diabetes, and the fiber they contain benefits digestion and lowers the levels of bad cholesterol. Fava beans are thought to affect the "pleasure center" of the brain and thus benefit mood. However, they should not be eaten by people who are treated with a mono amino oxidase inhibitor, or an enzyme deficiency that causes a very rare disease (hemolytic anemia) can develop.

One pod is 6 g.

One cup of raw pods of green fava beans contains (equals half cup dried fava seeds or 126 g) the following:

- 72 percent water or 110 calories g protein, 20 percent of DV
- 130 mcg of folate (a good level)
- 50 to 1,000 mg of levodopa. Fava beans in any form (green, fresh, or canned) are good for people with parkinsonism. It is also important for brain energy, memory, and sex drive.

Aside from high levels of iron, manganese, copper, and low level of sodium, beans are appreciated for their good taste, their nutritional value, and their high fiber content. Beans contain more nutrition pound for pound than do meats and dairy products and are high in vitamins, protein, folic acid, and magnesium (but no saturated fat). The folic acid content of beans is especially beneficial. If you consume 46 percent of your daily allowance of folic acid each day, you can decrease your risk for cardiovascular accidents. Remember that the folate in beans neutralizes the effects of homocysteine and thus reduces the risk for stroke and heart attack.

Dry fava beans (anti cholesterol factor, half cup at a time) are soaked then made into paste with olive oil and other spices like pepper and garlic. Each gram is 1 calorie. One cup contains 173 calories; 13 g protein; 30 g carbohydrate (10 percent DV); 10 g fiber (40 percent DV); and it is high in thiamine, folate, and zinc. It is a daily main meal in Egypt in breakfast. Sometimes eggs are added to the paste and eaten with bread. It is high in protein and fiber, low in sodium, and has no cholesterol.

Whole Grains

A serving is one slice bread or 2 slices of reduced-calorie bread. Around 80 calories.

Whole grains are one of the most important foods on earth! They are surrounded by (an inedible) husk. Each seed has three layers. After you remove the kernel, you'll find an outer layer called bran, which contains fiber, vitamin B, niacin, magnesium, zinc, and phosphorous. The middle layer, which is called the germ, is thin and contains no fiber, vitamins, or minerals. The thick inner layer, endosperm, is high in carbohydrates and protein but very low in vitamins and minerals. Here are some examples of whole grains and whole grain foods:

Buckwheat
Oatmeal
Popcorn
Whole grain tortillas and whole grain pasta
Bulgur
Brown rice
Wild rice

Refined Grains
Eat them when you have no other choice.

Refined grains, which lack bran, are low in fiber, iron, minerals, and vitamins but may be enriched with added nutrients. Unless the package label says "whole grain," you can assume that the respective food item contains refined grains. Here are a few examples of refined grains:

White bread
White rice
Couscous
Pasta
Some cereals, such as cornflakes
Flour tortillas
Fast-food bread and buns

Eating grains is good for those with diabetes. Research indicates that people who obtain their protein from grains and beans have a relatively lower risk for diabetes and heart attack. Studies have shown that overweight people who eat whole grains and beans had a lower incidence of cardiovascular disease than people who ate meat. Whole grains contain protein but are deficient in some essential amino acids. However, eating a combination of beans and whole grains, brown rice, or corn supplies a complete protein without saturated fats. Whole grains improve insulin sensitivity because they are high in magnesium, decrease the risk for gum disease, decrease the levels of bad cholesterol, and relieve constipation because they contain fiber.

If you eat grains, beans, grapes, and olive oil and reduce your consumption of saturated fats, you will reduce your risk for stroke and cardiovascular disease. Guaranteed! Just ask the French and the Mediterranean farmers.

Celiac Disease

This allergy to gluten disease can occur at any age but usually occurs in the young or in those older than seventy-five years. Celiac disease, which can be mild, moderate, or severe results in the poor absorption of nutrients and damages the mucosa (the lining) of the intestines. If you have celiac disease, you must avoid wheat, rice, pasta, and related foods and should eat vegetables, fruits, meat, olive oil, fish, gluten-free bread, and gluten-free pasta. Be sure to ask your doctor to check your thyroid and liver functions and your blood sugar level if you have celiac disease.

The diagnosis is made by a history of first-degree relatives with the disease, low blood pressure, pale, weak, peripheral neuropathy due to vitamin B deficiency, bruises under the skin due to vitamin K deficiency, bone pain from osteoporoses. A blood test called the celiac disease profile is used to detect detrain antibodies associated with the disease. Check for muscle spasm due to calcium and magnesium deficiency.

For definite diagnosis, a biopsy of the proximal part of the small intestine, duodenum, or better the jejunum, the lining of the intestine is. Instead of the fingerlike mucosa, it looks flat.

The treatment is a gluten-free diet, no grains or flour.

Brown Rice: The Manganese Factor

Brown rice has several varieties: basmati, brown, long grain, and black. Processing determines whether the rice sold is brown or white. When you remove the husk of the rice grain, it's brown rice; when you remove the outer layer of brown rice, you have white rice. When compared with white rice, brown rice has almost the same amount of protein, carbohydrates, and fat; but it is higher in levels of about sixty other nutrients. Just as the nutritional value of whole grain bread is higher than that in white bread, brown rice is more nutritious than white rice because the brown layer of the rice grain contains the highest levels of fiber and nutrients.

White rice is often enriched with vitamins B1 and B3, as well as other vitamins, but not with magnesium. However, brown rice contains 84 mg of magnesium per 100 g (a comparable amount of white rice contains only 18 mg). Brown rice has a mild nutty flavor that may intensify during storage. For that reason, brown rice is more perishable than white rice. One-quarter cup of cooked brown rice contains the following:

218 calories (very high)
Manganese, 100 percent DV
Magnesium, 25 percent DV, 1.6 g of fat.
No saturated fat
No cholesterol
No sodium
45 g of carbohydrates (12 percent of the daily value). Eat half or one-third cup at a time
3 g of fiber or 14 percent DV
4 g of protein

Vitamins B1, B2, and E, zinc, copper, and manganese. Now let's identify the differences between brown and white rice. Brown rice contains higher amounts of manganese, magnesium, riboflavin, and selenium than those found in white rice. If you eat one cup of cooked brown rice, it contains almost 50 to 60 percent of your daily allowance of manganese, which is very important in the synthesis of fatty acids and in the production of energy. It is important in converting protein and carbohydrates to energy, for nerve function and sensate perception, and an essential part for some antioxidant enzymes.

White rice does not provide most of those benefits, so brown rice is a more healthful choice. Brown rice contains selenium, magnesium, riboflavin, and fiber, which lower the levels of bad cholesterol. It facilitates weight loss; relieves constipation; and protects against hemorrhoids, chronic anal fissures, diverticulitis, and diseases of the blood vessels.

When you change your refined brown rice into white rice, you lose the benefit of the oil contained in brown rice, which helps to decrease the levels of bad cholesterol, and you also lose the good fatty acids in brown rice. Although white rice and brown rice contain the same calorie count weight for weight, white rice lacks protein and certain essential nutrients that are found in brown rice.

Magnesium, which is present in brown rice, is good for bone health. It usually precipitates on the surface of the bone and is reabsorbed when needed. This layer of magnesium can be very beneficial if you are ill or unable to consume a balanced diet. Magnesium also increases the level of nitric oxide in the bloodstream as do red and black grapes and red wine. It induces relaxation of small blood vessels, especially those in the heart, decreases fat deposits, and improves circulation to the cells. Magnesium is especially good for people with diabetes because it decreases insulin resistance; it decreases the levels of bad cholesterol and increases insulin sensitivity. It also decreases the risk of developing gallstones.

The extra fiber on brown rice binds the bile acids, which are fatty acids, and protects against cancer of the colon. Like most vegetables and fruits, brown rice contains phytochemicals, which exert an antioxidant effect. The magnesium and fiber in brown rice decrease insulin resistance, but white rice and pasta have the opposite effect.

We also know that magnesium is a calcium channel blocker, which means that it dilates blood vessels and exerts an antispasmodic effect, and it conveys more blood and thus more oxygen and nutrients to the cells. Brown rice contains manganese, fiber, beneficial oils, protein, complex carbohydrates, and about sixty other nutrients that include vitamins (such as thiamine) and minerals (such as potassium and niacin), all of which benefit the body and help it to use energy efficiently. Brown rice is also low in sodium.

Rye: Manganese, Selenium, Fiber, and Magnesium Factors

Rye is good for diabetes in one regular slice or two thin slices at a time.

This grain has a rich and hearty taste. Because its germ and bran cannot be separated from its stem, it is very nutritious. One cup of cooked rye contains

> 168 calories,
> Manganese (50 percent of the daily value),
> Fiber (35 percent of the daily value),
> Magnesium (20 percent of the daily value),
> Phosphate (22 percent of the daily value), and

Protein (20 percent of the daily value).

A thin bread slice is 0.7 oz or 52 calories, and a 1.1 oz slice is 83 calories. Rye contains a moderate amount of complex carbohydrates and is high in fiber, so it decreases insulin resistance. It absorbs water in the stomach and thus provides a feeling of satiety than other grains do. Some of the fibers in rye are cellulose, which absorbs bile acids in the intestines and reduces the risk for gallstones. Eating rye can decrease the level of triglyceride in the bloodstream, reduces bile acid absorption, and prevents constipation. It is one of the best grains for people who have diabetes.

There are two types of rye: processed rye and whole grain. Rye is rich in vitamins, particularly vitamin B, and protein. It is eaten as cereal, crackers, or bread.

Buckwheat: The Rutin Factor (anti retinopathy factor)

Buckwheat is grown in Russia, China, and Brazil in high amounts. It is also used as bread and tortilla. One cup or 170 grams contain the following:

583 calories (high)
22 g protein
6 g fat
48 g (one average slice) is 110 calories

It has the highest rutin in plant foods, which strengthens capillary walls, reducing the incidence of bleeding in hypertensive patients and reducing leaks in diabetic retinopathy.

CHAPTER 4

Fruits, Vegetables, Legumes, Nuts, Seeds, and Spices

A healthful diet is a nutritional mosaic that includes vegetables, fruits, oils and spices, legumes, nuts, and seeds, as well as the essential vitamins and minerals those foods contain. In this chapter, we'll review some of the most nutrient-rich choices in those food groups, many of which have been enjoyed as dietary staples for thousands of years.

Fruits, vegetables, and seeds have protein, carbohydrate, fat, vitamins, minerals, and micronutrients but in different quantities. The information here is available in other books or the Internet. My advice is just to tell you as a person entering the second chapter in life—after forty: what is good for you, I mean your situation, if you are underweight, overweight, diabetic, hypertensive, with eye disease, or just over forty without any disease for example. We need 1,200 mg calcium per day to help keep our bones healthy. Milk and cheese are good, but there are some people who can't tolerate both. I tell them that the nondairy, high calcium foods like figs, almonds and sesame seeds, or calcium fortified drinks like soy milk and orange juice. The second part of my work is to tell you which one of these foods is high in calcium. If you have diabetes, it has to have low glycemic load and low glycemic index; and if you have high blood pressure, to take the same foods with foods high in salt.

Remember when we say a fruit serving, we mean it has carbohydrate 80 to 100 calories, so a medium apple is a serving while a large apple is 1.5 serving.

Apples: A source of the Fiber Pectin
Serving size: a medium-size apple

Archaeological evidence indicates that apples were eaten by our ancestors in the Stone Age. An ancient symbol of love, beauty, and health, apples are among the most nutritious fruits. Eating apples and drinking apple juice have been shown to contribute to the overall good health and may offer protection against disorders as serious as heart disease, certain types of cancer, and the oxidative brain damage associated with aging and Alzheimer's disease. Apple pectin reduces bad cholesterol by binding to the bile fatty acids and removing them with the stool. This is an anticancer and decreases gallstones and constipation. It binds to the sugar in the stomach, slowing its flow and reducing the sugar absorption and improving the blood sugar level.

Because apples contain air, they float. One small apple weighs around 100 g, a medium-size apple weighs about 160 g, and a large apple tips the scale at about 200 g.

A medium apple contains

> 80 calories;
> about 90 percent water;
> 4 g of fiber (good);
> good amounts of vitamins A, C, K, and B; and
> beta-carotene.

Here are some facts about apples:

- Apples contain pectin, which lowers the level of bad cholesterol.
- There are more than 7,000 varieties of apples.
- Apples should be thoroughly washed and then eaten unpeeled.
- The color of the apple's skin indicates the type of antioxidants contained in the apple. Red apples, which are highest in antioxidants, have an oxygen radical absorbance capacity of 5,000.

Kiwifruit: The Vitamin C Factor

Kiwifruit is one of the most nutritious fruits. One ounce of kiwifruit contains the following:

- 46 calories
- High levels of vitamins C (50 percent of the daily value),
- E, and K
- 2.5 g of fiber
- Manganese, copper, and potassium (20 percent of the daily value)

Cherries: A Source of Vitamin C, Calcium, and Vitamin

Serving size: fifteen cherries

Cherries can be found in thousands of varieties that are tart or sweet. This delicious fruit, which is related to the plum, has been appreciated for thousands of years across the globe. Cherries are as nutritious as they are versatile. One cup of cherries contains 77 calories without pits and 50 calories with pits.

A cup of raw cherries (155 g) contains the following (each cherry is 8 g):

- 75 calories
- Fiber, 10 percent DV (daily value)
- Vitamin A, 39 percent DV
- Vitamin C, 25 percent DV
- Calcium, folate, and potassium

Pomegranates: A High Source of Antioxidants

Pomegranates contain one of the highest levels of antioxidants found in fruits. They are common in Asia and the Middle East; and in some cultures, they are a symbol of righteousness, good fortune, and abundance. A pomegranate that weighs 100 g (3.5 oz) contains

- 70 calories,
- 250 mg potassium
- a high level of pantothenic acid, which lowers the level of triglyceride,
- a high level of vitamin C,
- a high level of polyphenols, antioxidants, and
- Tannin, which is a potent anti-free radical agent.

Pomegranates can reduce the reaction of the foam cells that rupture under the lining of blood vessels, leak fat into the lining of arteries and cause a blockage in the injured blood vessel.

Reduce the systolic blood pressure level by working as antiangiotensin-converting enzyme (ACE) inhibitor. It has resveratrol like the black grapes. It is a good antioxidant and heart vessels dilator.

Bananas: Highest Source of Potassium in All Fruits

Banana has high calorie, high glycemic index when ripe and has high glycemic load. Serving size is a small or half medium-size banana.

Bananas contain tryptophan, which produces a calming effect and relieves emotional stress. Bananas are high in calories (a small banana contains 100 calories, a medium-size banana has 120 calories, and a large banana—about 135 g, has 140 calories). Ripe bananas, which can be recognized by the brown spots on their peel, have a high glycemic index and contain more calories than the partially ripened fruit, so they are a good snack for underweight people.

Bananas contain substances that can increase alertness and learning ability and may reduce depression. Eating a banana each day may reduce the risk of stroke. Bananas are good for the heart because of their high levels of potassium, vitamin C, and vitamin B, which relieves the symptoms of premenstrual syndrome (PMS). Because bananas are easily digested, they are antacid in effect and coats the lining of the stomach. They are a good snack for people with a stomach ulcer. Bananas are also good for people with diabetes. Because ripe bananas have a high glycemic factor, they are relatively high in calories and have a high glycemic load. Eat one small fresh banana or half to one-third of a large fresh banana at a time for a healthful snack.

A large ripe (no brown spots) banana contains

- all essential amino acids; zinc and minimal fats;
- 1 g of protein;

- 2.6 g of fiber; vitamin C (15 percent of the daily value);
- 850 mg of potassium, 20 percent DV, which is good for blood pressure and prevents stroke and those who take water pill Lasix; vitamins A, B2, B6, niacin, folic acid, magnesium, and iron;
- 30 g of carbohydrates as fructose, glucose, and sucrose
- (5 g glucose); and tryptophan, which is converted to serotonin (a neurotransmitter that improves depression and can help you to sleep).

Oranges: A Source of Vitamin C, the Highest Calcium in Fruits
Serving size: medium-size orange

Oranges are a very healthful food! They are far superior in nutritional value than other snacks such as french fries, foods sweetened with processed sugar, white rice, or sandwiches made of white bread. Because oranges contain fructose, which needs one and one-third of the insulin and fiber, they are not quickly digested. A small orange weighs about 100 g, a medium-size orange is 130 g, and a large orange is 180 g. Two 8 oz cups of orange juice provide folate, potassium, and 100 percent of the daily value of vitamin C. However, it is more healthful to eat the fruit of the orange, which provides fiber and other nutrients, than to drink orange juice.

A small (or 100 g) orange contains the following:

- 181 mg potassium
- 40 mg of calcium
- 50 mg of vitamin C about 83 percent water
- Essential amino acids

- 45 calories—a 100 g banana has more than double the amount of calories than orange
- 2.5 g of fiber
- Vitamin A, lutein, and beta-carotene

Orange Juice

The difference between orange juice and the raw orange cup is that the cup of juice has double the calories and has less fiber (0.5 g). The raw orange has 2.5 g fiber, which induces satiety.

You need two oranges to give one cup of juice.

Diabetics and overweight persons, take one medium raw orange; the orange juice is for young, growing, or active kids. Diabetics, drink half cup of the juice if you have signs of low sugar.

Limes: A High Source of Vitamin C and Potassium

The peel and the juice of limes add a burst of citrus flavor to beverages, sauces, meat or fish, jams, and desserts (key lime pie). One lime, two inches wide or 65 g, contains about 20 calories as well as vitamin C—20 percent of DV, and 1.7 g of fiber. Also, it contains iron, calcium, and vitamin A.

Lemon Juice, Vitamin C, and Potassium

Lemon juice is sometimes described as the *potassium and vitamin C factor*. It contains high levels of vitamin C and potassium but is low in calories, sodium, and fat. Lemon juice contains beneficial vitamins, minerals, and antioxidants that include calcium, magnesium, zinc, copper, manganese, selenium, vitamin K, vitamin C, niacin, and folate.

Pears: A Low Calorie Source of Fiber

Fresh pears are a healthful source of fiber (3 g of fiber per 100 g of fruit), and they are relatively low in calories (60 calories per medium-size pear). Pears contain a high level of vitamin C, which speeds wound healing and improves gum health, and antioxidants, potassium, iron, vitamin A, and selenium.

Watermelon: The Water, Vitamins A and C, and Potassium Factor
Serving size: half a cup balls of watermelon

Watermelon contains a high level of iron as well as vitamins and minerals equal to that of spinach. About 92 percent of the meat of a watermelon is water. Watermelon quenches thirst that's why it is called *water*melon. It is eaten in slices after the thick outer layer, which is usually green, has been removed. Watermelon is high in vitamins A, K, and C and in potassium. It has a high glycemic factor, so eat it alone or with low-calorie foods. One slice of watermelon that is about four by eight inches contains

150 calories (so it is not a good choice for dieters or diabetics);
201 g of water;
1 g of ash;
calcium, iron, magnesium;
potassium; manganese;
331 mcg of vitamin K (a very high level);
1046 mcg of vitamin A (a good dose);
27 mg of vitamin C, folate; and
niacin (a low level).

Remember these facts about watermelon:

- It is very nutritious, but it is high in calories. (Should be avoided in diabetics, or consumed in half a slice).
- The vitamin A in watermelon is good for night vision.
- The vitamin C in watermelon repairs cell wall damage. In addition, vitamin C is a water-soluble antioxidant that protects against free radicals and decreases the risk of heart disease and diseases of the blood vessels.
- It is high in potassium, which can lower high blood pressure.
- Its water content is high, so it causes satiety.
- It quenches thirst, so it is good for those with stomach problems or poor digestion.
- Its phytochemicals cause its rich colors.
- Because it is high in potassium, calories, and water, it is easily digested and absorbed.

Strawberries: The Vitamin C Factor

Strawberries is one of the highest in Vitamin C among all fruits. One cup halves or 45 g has 89 mg vitamin C or 150 percent DV.

It is high in magnesium and fiber, has low calorie, and is the best for diabetics. The serving size is four large strawberries or 1.5 cups. It has 90 percent water.

A large size strawberry of 1.5 inches is 18 grams and has 8 calories.

A medium size or 1.2 inches or 12 grams have 6 calories.

A small or 1 inch size or 8 grams have 4 calories.

A sliced one cup strawberry has 50 calories.

Diabetics and overweight people, strawberry is good for you, one cup at a time. It also contains 4 g fiber, which it is high. It's also high in magnesium, potassium, selenium, and vitamin C.

Calories and Fiber in Fruits

Let's compare the calorie count and fiber value of some of our favorite fruits:

1 cup of apple (1 medium-size apple): 120 calories and 3 g of fiber
1 cup of grapes: 100 calories and 1 g of fiber
1 cup of strawberries: 50 calories and 4 g of fiber
1 cup of fresh pears: 60 calories and 5 g of fiber

Avocado: The Potassium Factor

Avocado has potassium twice as much than banana of same weight, high calorie but mostly from good fats.

Potassium regulates the blood pressure. Avocado has the highest fat content in fruits, 80 percent unsaturated (60 percent mono unsaturated, 20 percent polyunsaturated).

A peeled half cup of avocado or 160 grams contain 200 calories, 75 percent from fat—high calories—but good for diabetics; it is from fat or carbohydrates of 10 g.

One 17 grams of avocado has high calories, 27 percent of DV, 14 g mono- and polyunsaturated fats, and 2.5 g saturated.

In summary, avocado is high in calorie but from unsaturated fats, which is good for diabetes. Fat doesn't require insulin to be metabolized. It is low in carbohydrates, high in oleic acid like olive oil. It reduces the bad cholesterol and increases the good cholesterol and has high vitamins E and C and as antioxidants.

Kiwifruit: The Third Highest in Vitamin C

Kiwifruit has 74 mg (a cup of strawberry has 89 mg and one lemon without seeds has 83 mg) of Vitamin C.

Serving size: one kiwifruit or 3 to 3.5 oz

The kiwifruit, which is one of the most nutrient-rich fruits, contains more vitamin C than an equal amount of orange. Kiwifruits may thin the blood to prevent clotting, and they seem to lower the level of fat in the bloodstream without adversely affecting the cholesterol level. These low-calorie fruits may also offer protection against the type of DNA damage associated with the development of cancer.

One ounce of kiwifruit contains

- 46 calories;
- 2.5 g of fiber;
- vitamin C (50 percent of the daily value);
- high amounts of vitamins E and K; and
- 20 percent of the adult daily value of manganese, copper, and potassium.

Grapefruit: Not for Everybody Factor
Serving size: half medium grapefruit

Tart grapefruit is low in calories. Grapefruit is an excellent source of many nutrients, and it appears to exert an anti-inflammatory effect. However, it is important to avoid grapefruit if you are taking any of several types of medication, such as a statin to lower your level of cholesterol, a drug to treat a psychiatric disorder, a medication to treat epilepsy, an antihistamine, or a calcium channel blocker. If your treatment includes one of those drugs, then consuming grapefruit can potentiate (increase the effect of) that drug and cause a toxic reaction. Grapefruit works almost like a medication in those cases. Otherwise, this citrus fruit is a healthful addition to the diet. One 100 g grapefruit contains

- 30 calories, which is good for weight control;
- water (about 90 percent);
- a high level of vitamin C, antioxidants, potassium, and vitamin A;
- fiber pectin (which lowers the level of cholesterol); and
- lycopene (for prostate health).

Papaya: A High Source of Beta-Carotene
Serving size: half papaya

Papaya contains more beta-carotene than any other fruit. A 3 oz serving of papaya has only 70 calories. Half of a papaya weighs about 150 g and contains

vitamin C 150 percent DV;
vitamin A, 30 percent DV;
Folate 13 percent;
potassium 10 percent;
water (about 90 percent);
calcium, iron, and boron; and
1.5 g fiber

Figs: A Source of Fiber and Calcium
(for people with lactose intolerance)
Serving size: two to three fresh figs (two-inch wide)

Fig fossils from more than nine thousand years ago attest to the enduring value of this nutritious fruit. The fig is mentioned in ancient recipes and is featured in the literature of antiquity. There are several varieties of figs (white, black, and green); and figs are grown in several sizes. They are high in fiber (which renders them an effective treatment for constipation) and a variety of essential nutrients. Four ounces of fresh figs has 44 calories, but an equal weight of dried figs contains 200 calories. Since raw figs has 80 percent water, each raw fig weighs as much as five dried figs.

Two figs, each two inches wide, contain 130 mg calcium, and high levels of potassium, iron, antioxidants, and vitamin k.

Each ten dried figs has 260 mg calcium, equals to a cup of milk, good for underweight people who are allergic to milk, as calcium supplement.
Fiber of 3 g works like a laxative.

Apricots: A Treat for Your Eyes
Serving size: four to five apricots

Apricots, which contain many nutrients that benefit ocular health, decrease the risk for macular degeneration, can help reduce cataracts, and may promote cardiovascular health by lowering the level of bad cholesterol.

One apricot contains 35 grams, 17 calories, and 0.7 gram fibers. The prunes' carbohydrates are table sugar type, which is low in fructose.

Three fresh apricots (about 100 g) contain the following:

- Water (about 86 percent)
- 48 calories
- 11 g of carbohydrates, 9 gm of glucose and sucrose (Diabetics be careful of the large amounts)
- 1,900 IU of vitamin A
- 1,000 IU of beta-carotene
- 89 mcg zeaxanthin and lutein
- 259 mg potassium
- Calcium
- A high level of tryptophan
- Fiber
- Lycopene

Pineapples: The Manganese Factor

Pineapples have the highest level of manganese in fruits. One cup has 91 percent DV. It has high glucose content. Avoid if diabetic.

Pineapples contain the following:

- A cup or 155 g or two slices size 3.5 inches wide and 0.75 inches thick has 75 calories
- 1.5 mg manganese—important to prevent osteoporoses like calcium, magnesium, and zinc

- 2.5 g fiber
- Magnesium and calcium 20 mg each
- Vitamins A and C
- It has 13 gm of sugar which is glucose and dextrose—both has high glycemic index

Coconuts: The Skin Healer
Serving size: one quarter cup, raw, unsweetened

It can give the organic virgin coconut oil. It is used for cooking or eaten fresh with salad and has 90 percent saturated fat, but the medium chain types don't change with cooking and don't behave like the meat saturated fat in raising the bad cholesterol.

It is grown in the tropical areas. Coconut water is used in juices; coconut oil comes from the dried meat of the seed. The oil is anti-inflammatory. When used as a cream, it works like alcohol, but with the cream advantage of being smooth and staying for a longer period. It is used for burns in poor areas; it is also used in soaps and massage oils. The virgin coconut oil has a shelf life of up to three years.

As food, it improves immunity, and it increases metabolism. It is anti-inflammatory and has antibacterial effect on the intestines.

Coconut: a cup, raw, unsweetened contain the following:

300 calorie (high calorie)
50 percent water
3 g proteins
26 g fat, 90 percent medium chain saturated fat

12 g carbohydrates

Beta-carotene

Phosphorous

Folic acid

25 mg magnesium

20 mg calcium

Iron

Coconut Water

It is the water inside the fresh coconut.

It is isotonic, like the human plasma, and is sometimes given intravenously.

It can rehydrate, can be used as a drink, and it is very nutritious. It has sugar and fructose, it is antibacterial, and can clear vesicles of chicken pox.

Grapes

Grapes, in particular the black and red grapes, go buy it tonight. It is the resveratrol Mediterranean life extender, the coronary vessel dilator factor. Serving size is fifteen grapes at a time (90 percent of the health benefit comes from the skin of the black and red grapes).

It is part of the Mediterranean diet. The darker the color, the more benefits. The red wine and the red grape juice are made from it.

Eating grapes may lower your risk for stroke because the flavonoids in that tasty fruit; this property is secondary to the resveratrol, which increases nitric oxide content in the intima of the heart and brain arteries. The skin of red and black grapes contains the highest concentrations of resveratrol, anthocyanins, and other potent antioxidants. Grapes increase the level of nitric oxide in the endothelium of the blood vessels (primarily those of the heart). They also increase blood flow, which transports oxygen and nutrients to the major organs of the body. For those reasons, people who drink red wine often tend to live longer and to have a lower risk for heart attack. Grapes supply the benefits of wine but not the risk for liver toxicity, pancreatitis, high blood pressure, and diabetes that is associated with drinking too many alcoholic beverages. Remember that grapes reduce the levels of bad cholesterol, decrease the level of triglyceride, decrease the level of total cholesterol.

Grapes increase the good cholesterol with its flavonoids and have the following:

- Protect against cancer of the breast, ovaries, and lung by reducing or stopping the rapidly dividing cancer cells.
- Contain resveratrol, a coronary artery dilator and a life extender
- Decrease the risk for chronic obstructive pulmonary disease (COPD) in smokers by decreasing the serum level of interleukin, which is an important inflammatory factor in the development of COPD.
- Contain antioxidants

Grapes exert three beneficial effects on blood vessels by decreasing blood clotting, dilating blood vessels, and decreasing blood pressure.

One cup (thirty grapes) or 150 grams have 100 calories. (Eat one-third cup or ten to fifteen grapes at a time.) It has 35 to 50 calories, which is good for diabetics because it has low glycemic load.

Potassium, 7 percent DV (low amount)

Vitamin K, 30 percent DV (reduce if you take Coumadin)

Vitamin C, 30 percent DV

Copper, 19 percent DV (good for osteoporosis)

100 IU vitamin A

100 IU lutein

.5 g fibers

Raisins
Serving size: 1 ounce

Raisins, the iron and resveratrol factor, is good one hour before exercise in nondiabetics. In diabetics, it is good for low sugar symptoms. It has the resveratrol too, which has anticancer function, by decreasing or stopping the growth of cancer cells, mainly the prostate and the breast.

It is dried or dehydrated grapes—white, green, and brown in color.

It is 60 percent sugar, mostly fructose; it is high in calorie and good for underweight and hikers (half ounce in diabetic at a time). It has high antioxidants like the prunes; it has boron, which is good for osteoporosis.

It is also good for snacks because it is light to carry and easy to store.

It decreases teeth cavities by its oleanolic acid, which is antibacterial. When the table sugar/sucrose invites cavities, raisin has natural fructose, which inhibits cavities.

One quarter cup equals 1 oz of raisins (equals fifty raisins) contain

100 calories;

1.5 gm fiber;

1.2 gm protein;

potassium, copper, and fiber, over 6 percent DV of each; and calcium, 1 percent DV.

Guavas

Serving size: one to two guavas

Guavas have more lycopene (red color) than any fruit (other sources are red tomato, red peppers, and watermelon).

Lycopene has 100 times more antioxidant power than vitamin E; it is a carotenoid.

Serving size: one to two guavas

- It can be eaten raw or as juice.
- One fruit is 50 g without ash.
- 40 calories (good for diabetics)
- 3 g fiber
- 1.5 g protein
- 10 mg calcium
- 125 mg vitamin C (200 percent DV), ten times compared to an orange with equal weight
- 2800 mcg lycopene (very high)—it is anticancer and reduces cardiovascular accidents
- Guavas contain vitamins A and B

Raspberries: The Fiber Factor and Vitamin C
Serving size: one cup

Ten raspberries equal 20 mg and have 16 calories. A cup of raspberries contains (123 g) the following:

- About 65 calories
- Vitamin C, 40 percent DV
- 8 g of fiber, 33 percent DV (This is high.)
- 30 mg calcium
- 27 mg magnesium
- 120 mcg lutein and zeaxanthin (Good for the eyes.)
- It has 15 mg choline, which is important in memory, intelligence, and cognition.

Vegetables

Parsley: The Blood Detoxifier Factor (Low Calorie)

Parsley is found in the Middle East, Europe, and in the United States. In a suitable climate, it grows all year. This herb, which contains twenty types of vitamins and minerals, is often eaten to decrease the odor of garlic. It is a flavorful addition to soups, salads, and sauces. Parsley is used as a garnish for entrees and is often eaten with lemon, garlic, and other spices. It protects against cancer (especially cancer of the lungs) because it neutralizes carcinogens in the blood, and it is a natural diuretic. Two tablespoons of parsley supplies the following:

- 50 percent of the daily value of vitamins K and E
- 133 mg (20 percent of the daily value) of vitamin C, which exerts an anti-inflammatory effect—vitamin C helps to relieve

asthma, nourishes red blood cells, lowers blood pressure and the levels of bad cholesterol, and is good for people with diabetes. Because it is water soluble, vitamin C can be found in the blood and in the intestines.

- 20 percent of the daily value of vitamin A
- Fiber
- Folate—lowers the level of homocysteine, protects the lining of small blood vessels and reduces the risk for stroke, cardiovascular accidents, and peripheral vascular disease
- Iron
- Calcium
- A minimal amount of fat
- Niacin
- Vitamin B6
- Selenium
- Vitamin E
- 420 mcg (47 percent of the daily value) of vitamin A, which is fat soluble and good for the eyes
- A high level of oxalates (So you should not eat a large amount of parsley if you have kidney stones.)
- A high level of chlorophyll. The chlorophyll, plus the calcium, manganese, selenium, as well as other vitamins, and specific flavonoids, like glycosides, work as cancer killers and detoxifiers in the bowel and the blood. It can neutralize the carcinogens of cooked meat and fungus-infected grains.
  - Other green vegetables which has high chlorophyll is spinach and broccoli.

Tomatoes: A Source of Lycopene, Beta-Carotene, and Vitamin A

Tomatoes are really fruits, but they are usually thought of as a vegetable. The red color of ripe tomatoes reveals the high level of lycopene in this versatile vegetable. Lycopene exerts antioxidant and anti-free radical effects, lowers the level of bad cholesterol and protects against certain types of cancer (prostate or colon cancer). If you eat cooked tomatoes, you will absorb more lycopene.

Tomatoes have a low glycemic load and a low glycemic index, are low in calories, and contain beta-carotene and phytochemicals both of which are antioxidants. The tomato has one thousand culinary uses. Tomatoes are added to pizza, rice, and pasta; enjoyed as a flavorful juice or a tasty soup; and eaten fresh in salads. They are a primary ingredient in catsup. Used as a paste, a sauce, or a puree, they add color, flavor, and essential nutrients to cuisine across the globe. Please add fresh tomato to your breakfast, lunch, and dinner!

A plum tomato weighs 60 g.
A medium tomato, 2.5 inches in diameter, is 130 g.
Larger than 3 inches, it is 185 g.
A medium-size tomato is 22 calories (good for diabetics and overweight)
It has 1.5 g fiber.
It has vitamins C, A, and K or 20 percent of DV.
It contains 12 mg calcium, 14 mg magnesium, and 76 mcg lutein and zeaxanthin.

It has 1,600 mcg of lycopene. (Lycopene is the red color carotenoid. As we said, it is a hundred times antioxidant than vitamin E. And while vitamin C action is reduced by cooking, lycopene function is increased by cooking. Other sources of lycopene are red pepper, watermelon, and papaya)

Tomato Juice

- A cup is 243 g
- 93 percent water
- 41 calories (good for diabetics and overweight)
- Vitamin C, 74 percent DV
- Vitamin A of 21 percent DV
- Potassium, calcium, and folate, each 13 percent DV
- 660 mg sodium, 40 percent DV (avoid with high blood pressure)
- Some tomato juices are low in sodium.
- 22,000 mcg lycopene, an excellent content

Squash: Low Calorie, High in Vitamins A and C, and Mainly a Good Source of Fiber

Squash is an excellent source of fiber, which is good to lower cholesterol, improve constipation, and to slow down carbohydrate absorption. One hundred grams of squash has a very low glycemic index of 20 and contains these:

- 15 calories
- 3 g of protein
- 3 g of fiber, vitamin A, 300 percent DV, potassium, 8 percent DV

- 20 mg magnesium
- 18 mg calcium
- Manganese, 9 percent DV
- Vitamin C, 32 percent DV
- 2,500 mcg of lutein, and a high level of niacin, 8 percent DV

Squash like cauliflower, broccoli, sweet pepper, lettuce, and cucumber has good nutritional value, low calorie, low sodium, and improves satiety. It is also good for weight loss, high blood pressure, and diabetes.

Broccoli: The Colon Detoxifier Factor and Anti-Alzheimer's.

It removes aluminum from the colon. It is high in vitamin C and calcium and has low calories. It has the sulforaphane, which is antiviral, antibacterial, and anticancer (also present in cabbage, cauliflowers, and radish).

It is a real good and nutritious vegetable. It was brought by the Italian immigrants.

What is unique about this vegetable is its function on cancer; it is a detoxifying agent. It stimulates some enzymes to neutralize and reduce end product of the human hormone estrogen, which stimulates breast cancer formation and decreases the spread of the cancer in case it started. Also, it detoxifies other precancerous chemicals and can reduce cancer of the rectum and urinary bladder.

It can detoxify aluminum in the colon, preventing Alzheimer's disease, which is worsened or caused by aluminum brain deposits.

One cup chopped broccoli, which is 90 grams, contain the following:

- 39 calories, low calorie (good for diabetic and overweight)
- Vitamin C 135 percent DV
- Vitamin K 115 percent DV (avoid with the blood thinner warfarin and others)
- 45 mg calcium
- 20 mg magnesium
- Folate, 14 percent DV
- Vitamin A, 11 percent DV

As you can see, teach your kids to eat broccoli. To cancer patients at any stage, eat broccoli. It has the chlorophyll in high amount. For diabetics and obese, it has low calories and it improves constipation.

People with family history of Alzheimer's, eat broccoli.

Carrots: A Source of Vitamin A, Low Glycemic Load

Carrots, which have a high glycemic index but a low glycemic load, are rich in nutrients such as beta-carotene. They can be eaten fresh in soups, salads, and cake or with an apple. Don't eat too many carrots (one cup serving a day is best) because the liver converts beta-carotene to vitamin A very slowly and only in small amounts. Eating a diet too high in carrots can cause beta-carotene to be deposited under the skin, which then develops a yellowish hue. Carrots are a healthful food when eaten in a reasonable amount each day.

Carrots improve night vision, can prevent macular degeneration, may prevent cardiovascular disease, contain phytochemicals and beta-carotene, both of which exert an anticancer effect may help to prevent emphysema in smokers.

One cup (100 g) of fresh carrots contains the following:

52 calories
450 percent of the daily value for vitamin A
Beta-carotene
Antioxidants a high level of vitamin K
15 percent of the daily value for vitamin C
15 percent of the daily value for fiber
Vitamins B1 and B2 (good for the nerves)
Manganese
Folic acid
Little sodium and fat (good for diabetics in moderate amounts, as well as hypertensive and overweight patients).

Carrot has high glycemic index but with low calories (low glycemic load) and good to lose weight. Don't eat too much of it, take only few cups and not few pounds.

Corn: A Source of Ferulic Acid (a good antioxidant)
Serving size: 3 cups popped light popcorn

Ferulic acid, a phytochemicals that fights cancer, is higher in corn than in other vegetables. Its content increases by heating the corn.

Evidence suggests that in some regions, corn has been a cultivated crop for nine thousand years. One hundred grams of this nutritious vegetable has 86 calories and 2.8 grams of fiber. A medium yellow and raw corn (90 g) also contains

- vitamin A, 10 percent DV;
- folate, 10 percent DV;
- thiamine, 10 percent DV;
- vitamin C, 10 percent DV;
- 40 mg magnesium, 10 percent DV; and
- 400 mg potassium, 10 percent DV.

Popcorn serving size of three cups (high in fiber but high in sodium).

Two tablespoons equals 35 grams and gives five cups microwave popped.

Each five cups, popped, has the following contents:

150 calories
4 g of protein
4.5 g fiber (good number)
50 IU vitamin A
1,100 mcg lutein and zeaxanthin (good for the eyes)
450 mg sodium, 25 percent DV (This is high, so avoid if with hypertension)
50 mg magnesium, excellent for diabetics

Okra: A Source of High Vitamin K, Calcium, and Fiber and Has Low Calorie.

Okra is a nutritious vegetable that is low in calories and fat. Popular in the southern United States, okra is often eaten fried or in gumbo, a soup or stew that contains meat and vegetables such as bell peppers, onions, and celery and is served over rice. It is a healthful choice for people who have diabetes. One hundred grams or eight pods of okra contains

- 33 calories; a minimal amount of fat;
- 2 g of protein;
- 860 IU of vitamin A, 65 percent DV (for night vision and dry eye);
- Lutein, 60 percent DV (It is important for vision.);
- Vitamin K, 65 percent DV. (avoid with the blood-thinning warfarin, but take when you have subcutaneous capillary leaks from weak capillaries);
- Vitamin C, 35 percent;
- Vitamins B1, B2, B3, and B6;
- 57 mcg of foliate, 25 percent DV;
- 75 mg of calcium; and
- 3 mg fiber, 12 percent DV.

Eggplant: The Source of Fiber, Low Vitamin K, Low Calorie

This oval purple or white vegetable, which has a slightly bitter but pleasant taste, is high in fiber and low in calories. Eggplants are an ancient vegetable long appreciated for their distinctive flavor. They are high in fiber and rich in phytonutrients (and thus in antioxidants), and eating eggplant may lower the level of cholesterol. In America, sliced eggplant is often breaded and baked or fried. Three ounces (100 g) of eggplant contains 24 calories—good for weight loss, diabetics, and satiety.

Water (about 90 percent)
3.5 g of fiber

14 mg magnesium

Vitamin K, 4 percent DV (minimal effect on warfarin or Coumadin)

Asparagus: A Source of Rutin and Glutathione

Rutin strengthens arterial and venous capillaries. Glutathione is a body detoxifier.

In many areas of the United States, tender stalks of asparagus in the local farmer's market signal the advent of spring! Often steamed and eaten as a side dish, asparagus is also enjoyed as a soup, in salads, and (after roasting) as an appetizer. Asparagus strengthens capillaries and exerts a natural diuretic effect. Because asparagus is high in purine, which breaks down to form uric acid, it should be avoided by people who have gout, kidney stones, or kidney disease. Eating asparagus also causes strong-smelling urine (metabolized sulfur products) and may interfere with the action of blood-thinning medications.

It is second to orange juice in folate content.

It has the flavenoid rutin; it promotes capillary health and regulates its permeability. That's why it reduces leg edema, diabetic retinopathy leaks, and chronic venous insufficiency, as well as improves leg circulation.

It has glutathione, which has three amino acids; it works as a body detoxifier, antiviral, and raises immunity.

A cup of asparagus has these contents:

- Low in calories (25)
- Low in sodium
- High in antioxidants, such as beta-carotene, which is 20 percent DV

- High in vitamin K, 70 percent DV (avoid with Coumadin)
- 2.5 g of fiber
- 2.5 g of protein
- Vitamin A, 20 percent DV
- Vitamin C, 12 percent

Cucumber: A Source of Fiber, Vitamins A, C, and Calcium and Has low Calories

The cucumber, which is really a fruit, is added to salads, served as pickles, and used as a natural treatment for eye fatigue, swelling, heartburn, and gastritis. It is also thought to lower high blood pressure.

Cucumber contains very low calorie—fullness factor.

For diabetics and overweight, eat it with salad before you start the carbohydrates to fill up the stomach early (it reduces the flow of foods and give satiety by its size and fiber).

Again it is like squash, cauliflower, tomato, and sweet pepper; it is good for weight loss. They have low sodium, high potassium, and all vitamins and have a low glycemic load.

A medium cucumber contains vitamin A, 13 percent DV or 650 IU, 40 mg calcium, vitamin C, 27 percent DV or 16 mg, 430 mg potassium, 10 percent DV.

Green Sweet Peppers: Low in Calories and Help Prevent Against Infection

Sweet green peppers also protect against tooth decay, help to relieve diarrhea, and improve digestion. However, they should be avoided by people with a stomach ulcer. A 100 g serving of sweet green peppers contains 20 calories, vitamin B6 (17 percent of the daily value), vitamin C (100 percent of the daily value).

Overweight and diabetics, eat sweet pepper with salad daily. It has little calories.

Cayenne peppers are small, red, and very hot. These peppers, which are antioxidants that contain capsaicin, can stop the itching and pain of peripheral neuropathy by depleting the levels of certain neurotransmitters.

Dietary Sources of Potassium

We need 4,700 mg of potassium daily. This essential mineral lowers high blood pressure and protects against stroke and heart disease. The foods and beverages listed below contain potassium in the following amounts:

- Dried apricots have 1,850 mg per 100 g
- 1 medium-size banana (100 g), 1,400 mg
- 1 cup of orange juice, 430 mg
- 1 cup of winter squash, 432 mg
- ½ cup of spinach, 430 mg
- ¼ cup of cantaloupe, 360 mg
- 1 cup of skim milk, 360 mg

Potassium reduces the blood pressure, protects the bones, and keeps the blood pH stable.

Leafy Green Vegetables

Examples of these vegetables are lettuce, spinach, fresh mint, fresh oregano, sage, cabbage, and turnip greens.

All are high in protein, fiber, phytochemicals (vitamins A, C, folate, and lutein); they are low in calories and fat.

Lettuce: The Chromium Factor

It stabilizes blood sugar and good for anybody—low weight, overweight, diabetics, and obese.

The chromium factor is in romaine lettuce (iceberg type has less nutrition).

Most used is romaine lettuce; also, it is the more nutritious.

And the greener the leaves the better.

A cup of lettuce contains 8 calories, which is good for dieting and for diabetics. It also has 1 gram of protein, high in potassium, phosphorous, vitamin K (50 mg), C, and folate. It is very high in beta-carotene (1,600 mcg) and lutein (1,100 mcg). In my opinion, the most important content of romaine lettuce is chromium (high content), which stabilizes blood sugar by helping the insulin push the glucose inside the cell to be utilized. The world's healthiest food ranked as a source of chromium is romaine lettuce, a one serving of two cups contain 13 percent of DV of chromium and ranked excellent since you can eat large amounts and at any time although one cup of onion has 20 percent of chromium DV. It is considered very good. Tomato cup contains 7 percent DV and is considered very good too.

Spinach: The Iron, Vitamin A, and Folate Factor

A rich source of iron of 2.7 mg or one cup contains

- vitamin K—181 percent DV,
- vitamin A—56 percent DV,
- manganese—14 percent DV,
- vitamin C—14 percent DV, and
- Folate—14 percent of DV.

It is a healthy food, good for diabetics and dieters.

Other Vegetables

Onions: The Chromium Factor

It is rich in sulphur-containing compounds, which is responsible for its smell and health benefits like cholesterol reduction and heart attacks, when combined with garlic. It has quercetin, which is an anticolon cancer.

Onion is high in chromium, which helps control the blood sugar and is high in vitamin C.

It also has vitamin B1, B6, and folate.

The green onion or scallion has more vitamin C and fibers.

Garlic: The Cholesterol-Reduction Factor
Serving size: four to five fresh cloves

Take before sleep to avoid the bad smell. Pills and cooked garlic have less action.

Garlic is one of the most nutritious spices. It has a delicious flavor but an unpleasant smell.

Fresh garlic leaves are rarely eaten; instead, the heads of the garlic plant are consumed. Each head consists of about twelve cloves. One of the most beneficial spices of garlic are the following:

- Prevents platelet clumping (aggregation)
- Decreases the level of bad cholesterol
- Decreases the level of triglyceride
- Inhibits atherosclerosis
- Reduces the level of homocysteine
- Exerts anticancer, antibacterial, antiviral, and antifungal effects
- Improves the level of blood sugar in people with diabetes
- Contains antioxidants
- Can be consumed in tablets or capsules that have no odor
- Improves immune system function
- Contains methylallyl trisulfide, which dilates blood vessels and lowers high blood pressure
- Contains the amino acid allicin, which is responsible for the spiciness of the raw garlic, which can give the other sulfides (sac and ajoene)
- Is not affected by cooking and also comes in pills

Dry Fruits with One Seed

Nuts: The Good Fat Factor
Serving size: half ounce for most nuts

Nuts are a very available source of multiple essential nutrients. A suitable addition to any meal, their nutritional value is appreciated worldwide. The term *nuts* usually refers to tree nuts such as peanuts, Brazil nuts, walnuts, almonds, hazelnuts (sometimes called filberts), pecans, coconuts, chestnuts, hickory nuts, cashews, macadamia nuts, pistachios, pine nuts.

Nuts are high in protein and fat. Eating only 1.5 oz of tree nuts daily (in conjunction with a diet that is low in cholesterol and saturated fat) may reduce the risk for cardiovascular disease. When they are eaten as a snack, nuts are usually roasted and shelled and may be salted. Because they are high in calories, they should be eaten in moderation. Nuts are also high in protein and good fats. Let's look closely at the nutritional value of a few favorite varieties of peanut—the source of phytosterol and beta-sitosterol—the cholesterol factor, and resveratrol for heart health.

One ounce or 30 g has the following:

> 13 percent DV of protein or 6.7 g
> 6 g carbohydrate or 2 percent DV
> 2.3 g fiber, 8 percent DV
> 14 g total fat (it has phytosterols)
> 2 g saturated fat, 10 percent DV
> 12 g unsaturated fats (the good ones)

The best thing in peanuts is that it has two sterols:

- Phytosterol (40 mg per ounce)—it is also high in soybeans and corn oil; it decreases absorption of fat in the intestine and reduces cholesterol. It is the cholestatin sold as OTC drug (if you can't tolerate the statins, try it with garlic pills).

- Beta-sitosterol—it decreases the absorption of cholesterol in the intestine, promotes prostate health by decreasing its size in benign enlargement, anticancer, improves immunity, and it works like an insulin stimulant.

Peanut Butter

It's high in calories but very nutritious. Peanut and peanut butter are good for athletes, the underweight, and common in poor areas.

It is the paste made from ground and roasted peanuts.

One cup has 1,520 calories. Take it in a teaspoonful at a time unless you are underweight.

So take one tablespoon at a time if you are active. You can take a tablespoon or 15 grams if you are not diabetic or obese.

Two tablespoonfuls of peanut butter contain the following:

- 190 calories (very high and is good for the active, young, and runners)
- 8 g protein (high and good for the poor to replace meat)
- 15 g fat, 2.5 g saturated only, the rest is mono- and unsaturated, the good one with 25 percent DV
- 2.6 g fiber
- Manganese, 30 percent DV
- 50 mg magnesium, 10 percent DV
- Niacin, it has folate and zinc

In larger quantities, it is good for marathon runners and is common in poor areas since it has high protein, fat, and calories. Some people do not carry it in their house since it is tasty, and kids like it a lot; it can result to obesity since a cup supplies over 1,500 calories.

Brazil nuts: The Highest Source of Selenium in All Foods

Selenium enables many enzymes to work as antioxidants, and Brazil nuts contain many times more selenium than any other nuts. Selenium exerts an anti-free radical, antiaging, and anticancer effects.

One ounce or 28 g or six to seven nuts
820 mcg selenium, 2,000 percent of DV
180 calories with 170 calories from fat
a high level of protein
a high level of fiber, vitamin E, iron
magnesium, 35 percent daily value

Macadamia Nuts: High Total Fats But With a High Source of Monounsaturated fat.

Its total mono- and polyunsaturated fats equals olive oil, which is 90 percent of their fat content. Macadamia nuts, which are native to Australia, are very healthful for people, but they are toxic for dogs. These pleasant-tasting nuts are very nutritious. They are high in fats and calories, but they contain no cholesterol. Monounsaturated fats are good to reduce the cholesterol.

One ounce of macadamia nuts has these contents:

- 180 calories (high calorie)
- 20 g of fat, 2 to 3 g of which is saturated fat (It is high but 90 percent of it is good fat. Just eat half ounce at a time or less unless you are underweight.)
- No sodium

- Vitamins A, B1 (thiamine), B2 (riboflavin), and B3 (niacin)
- Manganese, calcium, magnesium, and potassium
- 2.5 g fiber

Cashews: The Copper Factor

Cashews, which are native to Brazil, are from the same family as poison ivy. Cashew nuts have a pleasant, delicate flavor and are very nutritious, but they are high in calories and saturated fat. Cashews are never sold in the shell, which contains powerful irritants. Roasting shelled cashews at a very high temperature destroys any oil that might have been transferred to the nuts. Like peanuts, cashews can cause an allergic reaction that can be severe in some children.

One ounce of cashews (fourteen pieces) has the following contents:

- 140 calories
- 12 g of fat (3 g of saturated fat; 21 percent of the adult daily requirement)
- Copper, 35 percent DV
- Magnesium, 35 percent DV
- 4.5 g protein

It has fiber and high monounsaturated fat, which increase good cholesterol.

Pistachio Nuts

Pistachios are nutritious with low sodium and have low saturated fat.
Pistachio nuts are high in total fat content but low in saturated fats, so they are a healthful snack. Pistachios contain phytosterols,

which are substances that may lower the level of cholesterol in the bloodstream. One ounce of shelled pistachios or fifty kernels contain the list below:

- 160 calories
- 14 g of fat (total)
- 1.2 g of saturated fat (8 percent of the daily value)
- 3.4 g of fiber
- High levels of potassium, calcium, and magnesium
- Low level of sodium

Almonds: Highest Magnesium in All Seeds
(90 mg per one ounce—the magnesium factor)

Almonds, which have a delicate flavor, enhance many foods from salads to entrees, and they are also enjoyed as a snack. They may exert an anticancer effect. Because almonds are high in calories and fats (as well as in nutrients), be sure to eat 1 oz—and not 1 lb—of almonds at one time.

A cup (100 g) has the following:

- Manganese, 120 percent DV
- Calcium, 52 percent DV
- Vitamin E, 87 percent DV
- Copper, 52 percent DV

One ounce is twenty-two kernels and 168 calories. A kernel is 1.2 g and around 8 calories, mostly from the good fats.

Almonds contain the following:

- Vitamin E, alpha-tocopherol type (It is an antioxidant and can cross the cell wall since it is fat soluble, not like vitamin C, which is water soluble, and stays outside the cell. Vitamin C can recharge vitamin E if it is oxidized.)
- Polyunsaturated fats (It lowers the bad cholesterol, it has the phytosterols and the beta-sytosterol.)
- Vitamin C
- A high level of magnesium, which is healthful for people with diabetes
- Calcium

Almond is good for diabetes; it has a small content of complex carbohydrate with fiber and high magnesium but has high glycemic load, so eat five to eight seeds as a snack.

Walnuts: The Best Good Cholesterol Factor
(Just like niacin but cheaper and without the flushing.)

One cup of English walnuts or 117 grams contain 750 calories—that's why it is eaten half ounce at a time.

Black walnuts have less phytosterols but are higher in arginine and selenium and fiber.

It has all the benefits of nuts—high protein, high unsaturated fats, low carbohydrates, and one additional benefit—it increases the good cholesterol. An Australian research showed that eating one ounce or five to six nuts per day increases good cholesterol by 30 percent (as good as niacin but without flushing and with twenty other nutritional factors). It also reduces the bad cholesterol, it has fibers, it gives satiety, and it decreases its rate of absorption.

When you eat extra walnuts, reduce the saturated fats (from meat and milk products) to keep your weightin check.

One ounce has these contents:

- 185 calories (Eat half ounce at a time. Unless you are underweight, you can eat more.)
- 2 g fiber (The black walnut has 12 g fibers.)
- 18 g fat with 2 g saturated (good)
- 48 mg magnesium
- Vitamin E

Note:

Most diabetics, if not all, has low good cholesterol. And remember, good cholesterol level is important and soon may be declared more important than bad cholesterol on their effect on the heart, so any diabetic who doesn't take four to six halves walnuts per day, at least five days a week, and has no problem in eating it, please start now (if you don't eat walnuts, you are nuts).

On the other hand, most of people who are overweight think that eating nuts is nutritious, and it has nothing to do with weight. Nutritious yes, but for weight increase, it is a big unrecognized factor.

Sesame Seeds: A Source of Vitamin B1 (Thiamine), Copper, Manganese, and Vitamin E

For more than five thousand years, sesame seeds have served as a nutritious and flavorful addition to foods. It is a source of oils used for cooking and an appealing garnish. The color of sesame seeds ranges from white to black. In antiquity, these tiny seeds were thought to be a source of beauty, vigor, youth, and strength. Used today in foods, skin treatments, and body oils, they are appreciated for their versatility for their light, pleasant, nutlike flavor and for their crunchy texture. They are often ground into a paste called tahini, which is used in Middle Eastern dishes such as hummus and in sweets like halva.

One ounce of sesame seeds has these contents:

150 calories
130 calories from fats mg of calcium (a very high level) or 20 percent DV
1 mg of copper or 35 percent DV
Manganese, 35 percent DV (high level)
79 mcg of folate (high level)
100 mg of magnesium, 25 percent DV
15 gm of fat, 12 gm mono- and polysaturated
4 g of protein
6 g of carbohydrates
2 g of fiber
Zinc (20 percent of the daily value)
Phosphates (20 percent of the daily value)
Vitamin B1 (thiamine) or 50 percent of the daily value

However, sesame seeds are potent allergens that can cause a severe allergic reaction in some people. The reaction may be mild hives but may give anaphylactic reaction with severe and fatal complications.

Grape Seeds

Grape seed extract is a good antioxidant. It has a granulated proanthocyanidins; it has twenty times more antioxidant value than vitamin C and fifty times more than vitamin E. It is good, and its main effect is on small arteries and veins. It strengthens the capillaries, reducing the leak in retinopathy and chronic venous insufficiency when the venous valves are damaged. The second main function is for Alzheimer's and memory loss.

It also has a natural antihistamine effect and is good for eczema.

It comes in capsules, tablets, or liquid.

The dose is 500 mg daily.

Pumpkin Seeds and Squash Seeds:
The Benign Prostatic Hypertrophy Factor

Eating roasted salted pumpkin seeds and squash seeds can help to prevent benign prostatic hyperplasia. One cup (227 g) of either of those seeds contains 1,200 calories, so you should not eat more than 1 oz (a half ounce is even better) at one time.

One ounce of pumpkin seeds or squash seeds contains the following:

- 2 g of water
- 160 calories
- 10 g of protein
- 13 g of high monounsaturated fat (good one)
- 4 g of carbohydrates

- 1 g of fiber
- 3 mg zinc (It may be the reason that pumpkin seeds are good for enlarged prostate.)
- Manganese, 50 percent DV
- 100 mg of calcium, 10 percent DV
- 4 mg of iron, 25 percent DV
- 170 mg of magnesium, 23 percent DV
- 340 mg of phosphorous
- 230 mg of potassium
- 150 mg of sodium
- 120 mg of vitamin A

When compared ounce for ounce with other seeds, pumpkin seeds and squash seeds have the highest levels of fat, magnesium, phosphorous, potassium, vitamin A, iron, sodium (if roasted eat half ounce at a time), and calories (eat half ounce if over weight).

Flaxseeds: Ant breast Cancer Factor

This is highest in lignan or the plant type estrogen, which is an antibreast cancer factor, and the highest omega-3 in all seeds.

This is an interesting seed. It has a lot of benefits; it has vitamins, minerals, and trace elements. It also has high content of soluble mucilage and nonsoluble fibers. It also has low carbohydrate content. Thirty-three percent of its weight is oil, which has omega-3 and alpha-linolenic acid that can give the EPA and DHA the other components of omega-3 and the other two omega fatty acids.

Flaxseed has more omega-3 than any seed; it has 50 percent of its fat as omega-3. The next in content is pumpkin seeds.

One tablespoon of seeds—10 grams, is 55 calories (high, almost like sugar).

One tablespoon ground seed or 7 grams contain 32 calories, 1 g protein, 3 g lipids, 1.5 g omega-3, the anticardiac arrhythmia. It reduces cholesterol, blood pressure, eczema, and psoriasis.

It has lignans—the antibacterial, antiviral, and anticancer property—more than any seed or vegetable.

One of the most important content of flaxseed is the phytoestrogen, lignan, or the plant estrogen. It can block the estrogen receptors; it is antimitotic, reducing the risk of cancer of the breast, ovaries, and prostate.

Flaxseed has lignans twenty to eight hundred times than any other plant food, which contain lignans, like whole wheat and cabbage.

The flaxseed pill has no fiber and has minimal lignan.

Take one tablespoon ground seeds with juice daily—it has more lignans—then increase the dose.

Watermelon Seeds: The Iron and Zinc Factor

One ounce (roasted) contains

- 13 g fats, 3 g saturated;
- low carbohydrate;
- 130 calories;
- copper (20 percent of the daily value);
- zinc (25 percent of the daily value); and
- iron 14 percent DV.

CHAPTER 5

Herbs, Vitamins, Spices, Aboya Coffee, and Tea

Some of our favorite condiments and beverages have been used since antiquity to enhance diet and ensure or restore good health. Spices are aromatic herbs that have been used as flavorings and medications to treat disease, prevent illness, or ensure good health. For example, ginger can improve digestion and motion sickness; mace relieves colic and diarrhea; and cinnamon benefits digestion, relieves sore throat pain, and helps control sugar. Spices stimulate the flow of saliva and improve digestion, and those that are pungent can cause sweating. Some spices are cooling in effect; others provide a sense of warmth.

In this chapter, we'll examine the benefits of vinegar, coffee, tea, water, catsup, and several spices, all of which have multiple uses that are rooted in cultural heritage and tradition and have been validated by contemporary science as beneficial to our health.

Vinegar:the insulin helper factor.

Diabetics, if you don't remember anything in this book, it is okay but to forget vinegar, no; it is the most type of food, which is an insulin-sharpening factor (it increases the insulin sensitivity by 30 percent). Diabetics, please remember it. Add it to olive oil and salad, the Italian restaurants know that apparently.

Vinegar has been used as a flavoring, medicine, preservative, and cleaning agent for thousands of years. Vinegar forms when sugar ferments in the presence of air (aerobic fermentation). Vinegar contains vitamins C and A, magnesium, zinc, manganese, iron, potassium, a minimal amount of protein, a minimal amount of fat, and very few calories.

The prophet Mohammed used vinegar and recommended it as a dip for foods such as salad, olive oil, and bread. Vinegar is good for people with diabetes and those with a prediabetic condition. It can lower the level of blood sugar, lower the level of insulin in the bloodstream, and increase insulin sensitivity by up to 30 percent.

Add vinegar to your salad or take one table spoonful of vinegar before a meal. Don't forget that vinegar is extremely sour, so if you cannot tolerate its taste, be sure to combine it with food.

How does vinegar affect diabetes?
In people with diabetes, vinegar has the following action:

- It lowers the level of blood sugar because vinegar is high in acetic acid. Vinegar also delays the absorption of sugar from the intestines. Research has shown that if you take vinegar before a meal, your level of blood sugar will have decreased by 25 percent approximately one and one-half hours after that meal.
- Vinegar causes early satiety. Swedish researchers have shown that consuming vinegar diluted with water before a meal may reduce weight and curb overeating.
- It improves insulin sensitivity because it contains magnesium.

It also has additional uses:

- Reduces swelling after injury (it is even more effective than ice).
- Just apply a cloth soaked in vinegar over the injured area for few minutes.
- Has an antiviral effect.
- Can be used as a disinfectant.
- Increases the absorption of calcium, so you should take a calcium supplement with vinegar, lemon juice, or food that contains vitamin C.

Sources of vinegar include rice, apple cider, grapes, other fruits.

Wine vinegar, which has a grapelike flavor, contains flavonoids (antioxidants) such as resveratrol. Antioxidants neutralize free radicals and dilate the coronary arteries. However, oxygen reduces the effect of resveratrol, so you should buy small bottles of wine vinegar or use it quickly.

Rosemary: A Memory Factor

Rosemary, which is called the holy herb, helps memory. One teaspoon of rosemary contains 10 calories and 1.5 grams of fiber. Rosemary leaves are often used in wedding ceremonies to represent the wish to always remember that happy occasion.

Rosemary contains vitamin B6, folate, vitamin C, iron, calcium, magnesium, potassium, and vitamin A.

Adding rosemary to green tea creates a beverage that is good for memory and improves brain function. Remember that rosemary

- improves brain circulation,
- reduces high blood pressure,
- improves circulatory problems,
- prevents infection,
- is a decongestant,
- is an antitumor agent that may help prevent cancer, and
- relieves menstrual cramps.

Chamomile: The Nerve-soothing Factor

Chamomile reduces Alzheimer's and insomnia. Add it to green tea; its action comes maximum in ten minutes or less.

Chamomile, which induces relaxation and soothes frazzled nerves, is a plant with evergreen leaves and a single yellow flower. This flower produces deep blue oil that provides polysaccharides and imbues chamomile with its characteristic flavor. Add chamomile to tea flavored with honey, cinnamon, lime, or lemon for a delightful drink. However, chamomile must never be consumed during pregnancy or with milk. The best chamomile is grown in the Nile Delta in Egypt. Chamomile contains calcium, magnesium, manganese, potassium, vitamin A, tannic acid, and chamazulene acid

Chamomile is a mild sedative that soothes the nerves, a treatment for migraine and headache, and an effective mouthwash.

Chamomile relieves sunburn, diarrhea, gastric reflux, flatulence, irritable bowel disease, menstrual pain, and insomnia.

If you are emotionally stressed or worried and have a headache, brew a cup of green tea and add some chamomile.

Sage: The Word-Recall Factor

If you can remember the memory factor, add it to green or brown tea always.

Sage, which is from the mint family, was designated in 2000 as the Herb of the Year by the International Herb Association in Florida. Fresh or dried sage, which exerts a mild antimicrobial effect, is an anti-free radical agent that is often used in cooking. When brewed, sage releases a potent mustardlike astringent and warm aroma. Sage contains ten substances that benefit health, including camphor, tannin, carnosic acid, which and carnosol prevents brain aging and improves memory.

To prevent Alzheimer's disease, sharpen your senses, and improve your memory, drink a cup of tea with sage every day. Sometimes termed the *immediate-recall herb* or the *word-recall factor*, sage can be found in stores that carry spices and/or Middle Eastern foods. The genus name of this herb, which is *Salvia*, is derived from the Latin word meaning "to save."

Sage exerts an anti-inflammatory action; and its volatile oils contain antioxidants, flavonoids, and saponins.

It can be used as a mouthwash, and it stimulates digestion, decreases salivation, and contains an estrogen-like substance.

Cardamom: A Memory Factor

Cardamom is a vase dilator of small vessels. It can dilate the brain vessels and counteract the hypertensive effect of coffee.

The Indian spice cardamom improves memory. It dilates small blood vessels, including those in the brain and reduces the hypertensive action of coffee. The cardamom fruit is a capsule that contains seeds with a strong, pungent aroma caused by volatile oils, which account for 2 to 8 percent of the weight of the seeds. Covered by their protective pod, cardamom seeds can remain fresh for long periods. When compared with other spices, cardamom is expensive by weight. It is white, green, or black color.

Cardamom can be used as a breath freshener, a remedy for hiccups, a cure for stomachache, and an aphrodisiac.

As I mentioned before, dried cardamom improves memory and dilates small blood vessels when added to coffee (or tea). Just add four or six seedpods to enough boiling water to make two eight-ounce cups of coffee.

Thyme: The Intelligence Factor

Thyme is a memory builder. Feed it to the kids and all ages (If you want to be a doctor, eat zaatar, it is from oregano and thyme).

The Mediterranean spice thyme is used as fresh or dried leaves, flowers, or berries. It can be easily grown as a houseplant. Possibly, it has the highest antioxidant than all herbs and foods. In Lebanon, the families feed their kids with zaatar (mainly thyme) the day of examinations in the school so their kids can score better.

It contains antioxidants, which protect against nitrous oxide and help to inhibit platelet aggregation. Thyme can easily be grown at home. It is often combined with sesame seeds, salt, soy or olive oil, and sumac in a tasty mixture called zaatar that is added to bread, cheese, or hummus; eaten alone or with olive oil; added to tomato slices dressed with olive oil; or eaten on whole wheat bread with low-fat cheese, which is a good breakfast.

Facts on thyme:

- It is a relatively inexpensive spice.
- It improves memory.
- It is called the intelligence factor in the Middle East, where it is used in a spice medley called zaatar or *dokka*, which can be bought in most Middle Eastern food stores.
- It counteracts the effects of nitrous oxide, which is a free radical.
- It is an expectorant.
- It is an antibacterial and antifungal that is used in the mouthwash Listerine.
- It is an antispasmodic.
- Thyme is effective in the treatment of bronchitis, diarrhea, gastritis, and it improves appetite.
- It helps memory, especially when combined with other spices in a seasoning called zaatar or dokka, which can be purchased in Middle Eastern food stores.
- It contains a very high level of copper and manganese. When combined with sesame seeds, thyme provides even more copper and manganese.

One-fourth cup of thyme provides the following:

- 75 percent of the daily value of copper
- 35 percent of the daily value magnesium (which lowers high blood pressure, stabilizes the blood sugar level in people with diabetes, and protects against heart disease)

- Chromium (which, like magnesium, lowers high blood pressure, stabilizes the blood sugar level in people with diabetes, and protects against heart disease)
- Zinc, which is good for the eyes and immunity
- Tannic acid, which is important in brain function

Zaatar

Zaatar is a mixture of herbs that contains the highest level of antioxidants known. Eaten alone or as an accent to other foods, zaatar is almost a part of the daily diet in Palestine. Zaatar should be eaten by anyone who wants to excel. It has given Palestine its tens of thousands of medical doctors, pharmacists, and scientists who eat zaatar every morning (several times a day, like me).

Termed the *intelligence factor*, zaatar contains high levels of minerals, trace elements, vitamins, antioxidants, and it has very low calories!

It is a mixture of dried ground oregano or thyme leaves, sesame seeds, olive oil, and sumac powder. Zaatar is often eaten with tomato slices, olive oil, and cheese on bread. It can be mixed with olive oil and spread on any dough before it is baked, and it can be enjoyed at any time during the day.

The French have a diet that is high in red grapes, wine, beans, and meat; and perhaps because they eat those antioxidant-containing foods, as well as the type of protein in the beans, their incidence of heart disease is relatively low. Italians have a diet that is rich in olive oil, and although overweight or obesity might be common in that population, Italians tend to live to an old age, perhaps because olive oil is a life extender. The Eskimo diet is high in cold-water fish; and although Eskimos tend to be overweight, they live a long life, perhaps because of the high level of omega-3 fatty acids that they consume each day.

In the Palestine of my youth, we were poor. Our diet was low in meat and high in grains, olive oil, zaatar, and, (for three months a year in summer) grapes. In the winter, we often ate dried figs and raisins. Most Palestinians lived to an old age (ninety to one hundred years) until the 1960s when their diet changed. Their consumption of sweet confections—colas that contain high-fructose corn syrup and eating ice cream—is now high, and fast-food restaurants seem to be everywhere. The level of stress is also higher. Perhaps, as a combination of those factors, the lifespan of the Palestinian people has shortened, in spite of which they remain among the most educated people on earth, over 98 percent. *Education* has many meanings, but in Palestine today, all children complete the ninth grade. My mom used to say, "If you eat zaatar, you will be a doctor." That encouraged me, and now, I am a physician and a firm believer in the benefits of zaatar in helping me to achieve that goal. My people are all over the world: PhD, engineers, pharmacists, and doctors in a gulf state, the first nine kids in the class were Palestinians. Their friend said it is not that they are smart; it is because they eat zaatar. I always have zaatar in my home (in fact, around my house in the USA, I plant only thyme and peppermint, the leaves of which can be eaten fresh).

It is important to know that 100 g thyme, which is an ingredient in zaatar, has an oxygen radical absorbance capacity (ORAC) or total antioxidant capacity (TAC) of 160,000 when it is consumed as oil. One hundred g of red apples contain only

5,000 ORAC, and 124 g of red beans—a food that is very high in antioxidants—contains 14,000 ORAC. Calculate which has the better value and eat some zaatar! And don't forget that zaatar has sesame seeds, sumac, olive oil, and thyme.

Mint: The Intestinal Spasm Relaxing Factor

Mint is an aromatic herb with multiple uses. It's cool, pleasant flavor and medicinal value have been appreciated since antiquity.

Here are some facts about mint:

- It is a diuretic.
- It is used as an antiseptic mouthwash.
- It is used to treat stomachache and chest pain.
- Its aromatic oil is used in candy bars, sweets, breath fresheners, and perfumes, as well as in cigarettes to minimize the bitter taste of tobacco.
- It helps to burn fat.
- It contains traces of vitamins A, B, C, and E; zinc; folate; and potassium.
- Peppermint is the most popular type of mint.

Hibiscus

Hibiscus, a flowering plant grown in the Nile Delta, is often consumed in beverage form (especially as tea). Hibiscus is high in vitamin C and is caffeine free. It has an astringent flavor and shows deep red color in a glass cup. It is used for respiratory problems and to reduce fever.

Fenugreek: The Insulin Stimulator Factor

Fenugreek is an herb that exerts a Glucotrol-like effect. It is beneficial for people with diabetes.

Here are some facts about fenugreek:

- It has a strong smell when secreted in the sweat that is not pleasant.
- It has been used for thousands of years for diabetes and breast milk production.
- The fenugreek plant has green leaves and yellow seeds.
- Fenugreek is one of the herbs added to curry.
- In Arabic, the word for fenugreek is *hulba*.
- Fenugreek is grown in Mediterranean countries.
- Fenugreek is high in fiber, which reduces the level of blood sugar. It delays sugar absorption.
- It is a bulk-forming laxative.
- It contains volatile oils.
- It contains alkaloids (a type of protein such as L-tryptophan) that stimulate the pleasure center in the frontal lobe of the brain and induce relaxation.
- Fenugreek can reduce calcium oxalate crystals in the urine.
- It can reduce the size of kidney stones.
- It exerts an anti-inflammatory effect.
- It contains an estrogen-like substance.
- Its high fiber content decreases the levels of bad cholesterol and triglyceride.

In the Middle East, fenugreek is used to treat two conditions:

- Diabetes (adult onset as well as juvenile)—because fenugreek reduces the blood sugar level, sometimes enough to cause hypoglycemia (a low blood sugar level). If you like the taste of fenugreek and you have diabetes, consult your doctor about how much of that herb you can safely consume. Start by consuming a small amount of fenugreek and then see whether your doctor wants to reduce the dosage of any of your medications.
- Failure to produce breast milk. Fenugreek is a galactagogue
- (a milk stimulator) in women who are breast-feeding.

A quantity of ten tablespoons of fenugreek weighs 100 g. One tablespoonful of fenugreek contains the following:

35 calories
1 g of fat
6 g of carbohydrate
3 g of protein
2.5 g of fiber
25 mg of sodium
Vitamin A
Vitamin C
Biotin
Folate
Vitamin B6
Vitamin B12
Vitamin D
Calcium
Iron

The usual dosage of fenugreek is 400 mg in capsule form, three times per day.

Do not consume more than 6 g of fenugreek per day.

Adverse effects caused by fenugreek include an increase in blood thinning and thus an increase in bleeding, but that effect is rare.

Coffee: The Most Addictive Drug On Earth
(Caffeine, Cocaine, and Nicotine Are of the Same Family)

Coffee was used in Egypt more than two thousand five hundred years ago. According to tradition, the discoverer of coffee was a shepherd who noticed that in his flock of goats, those that had eaten a local red berry were lively and active. When the shepherd consumed a few of the berries, he felt their benefits. He described his discovery to his superior, who obtained some of the berries and used them to make a drink that he served to his followers. The worldwide coffee industry blossomed from that humble beginning. Today, we know that the caffeine in coffee increases energy and concentration.

Caffeine is found in coffee beans, tea leaves, and cola nuts.

How Does Caffeine Work?

Caffeine exerts its characteristic effects by binding to the brain receptors for sleep. It stimulates dopamine secretion in the frontal lobe of the brain, which produces a sense of pleasure. In addition, caffeine increases short-term memory and improves memory overall. Unfortunately, its effects mimic those of a minidose of heroin in some ways. When the stimulatory effects of caffeine wear off, we feel depressed and fatigued, and we start looking for more coffee. If you drink coffee regularly and you forgo it for twenty-four hours, you will feel tired and will have a headache and muscle pain, which are symptoms of withdrawal. Caffeine is the most frequently used drug in the world, and it has the most addicts.

How Much Caffeine Is in a Cup of Coffee?

The amount of caffeine in a cup of coffee depends on the size of the cup and on the type and concentration of the coffee. Usually, an 8 oz cup of coffee contains 100 mg of caffeine, so drinking three cups a day is okay. Consuming more coffee than that amount daily may produce restlessness, gastric irritation from excess stomach acid, and even gastroesophageal reflux. If you consume coffee (and hence caffeine) with a nonsteroidal anti-inflammatory drug such as ibuprofen (Motrin) or naproxen (Naprosyn), you may experience palpitations and an increased heart rate. Here is information about the caffeine content of a few popular beverages:

> Two ounces of espresso contain 100 mg of caffeine, and 12 oz has 600 to 1,000 mg or more of caffeine.

Other caffeine-containing drinks in 12 oz portions have the following caffeine content:

> Brewed coffee: 150 mg (raises the blood pressure)
> Instant coffee: 100 mg
> Decaffeinated coffee: 5 mg (has low caffeine, but with the same nutrients)

Black tea: 40 mg
Green tea: 10 mg (reduces the blood pressure)
White tea: minimal amount
Coke (12 oz): 30 mg
Energy drinks: 40 mg

Benefits of Coffee Consumption

Coffee offers several benefits if you don't drink too much of it and if it does not interfere with the effects of your medications. Theophylline increases the effects of coffee. For most adults who do not have a stomach ulcer or gastric reflux, drinking three 8 oz cups of caffeinated coffee per day is okay. A cup of coffee contains minimal calories if no sugar is added and skim milk is used.

Here are some facts about the benefits of coffee:
It improve the motor function and improve coordination with a reasonable caffeine dose(120 mg)

- It can improve gout.
- It increases short memory and improves memory overall.
- It induces a sense of pleasure.
- It is an antioxidant (but consuming antioxidants in fruits, which contain necessary nutrients, is more beneficial).
- It is a mild diuretic.
- It increases alertness.
- It increases the accuracy of performing tasks such as typing.
- It sharpens vision.
- It contains magnesium, which is helpful in diabetes.
- It is good (especially in the decaffeinated form) for people with diabetes.

Coffee consumption is also associated with adverse effects, most of which develop after two or three cups per day have been consumed. Remember that coffee should not be drunk by people with cardiac disease or those who have had a myocardial infarction,

Coffee can cause a miscarriage in women who drink it during the first three months of pregnancy. It can have these side effects:

Reduction in fine motor function and muscle irritability and disturbed coordination when taken in high doses. Or in withdrawal cases

- An increased heart rate
- Dehydration
- Constipation
- Diarrhea
- Gastric irritation
- Gastric reflux
- High blood pressure (by constricting the small blood vessels under the skin)
- Pallor
- A temporary decrease in vision in people with retinopathy

People who drink four to five cups of coffee daily may experience restlessness, insomnia, and/or depression.

Some psychiatry hospitals and doctors' visits are related to unrecognized caffeine toxicity or withdrawal. The toxic dose is 60 mg per pound for a 200 lb person. Twelve grams are toxic and may be fatal; smaller doses may do the same.

For infants a 200 mg is toxic, they can't handle coffee.

To avoid caffeine problems and to extend your life, take the farmer's son's coffee.

The Farmer's Son's Coffee (Aboya Coffee or My Father's Coffee)

We can't stop Americans from drinking coffee, although CNN's Sanjay Gupta, MD, mentioned that if you stop drinking coffee, you will add one year to your life, and I agree. If coffee is truly beneficial to health, then why is this true? Some people add cream to their coffee, which is high in saturated fat, or they may add an artificial sweetener that can cause health problems.

Here are some facts about the effects of coffee:

- It increases blood pressure because it constricts under the skin capillaries.
- It causes dehydration.
- It can cause osteoporosis from frequent urination and increasing the calcium loss. Acute toxicity—if you consume 7 to 12 g of coffee in few hours, then caffeine toxicity, which is characterized by headache, chills, fever, anxiety, dizziness, nervousness, tremors hallucinations, and later, seizures and is sometimes fatal.

When semicomatose patients who have overdosed on alcohol are admitted to the emergency department, they are usually incoherent and sleepy, but they regain consciousness; immediately after a 1 g intramuscular injection of caffeine, they become more alert and can breathe more easily.

Chronic caffeine toxicity gives anxiety and psychoses and (RVRN) dementia.

Here is my recipe that can make your coffee a more healthful beverage. To prepare 8 oz of caffeinated coffee: add soy milk fortified with calcium instead of milk or cream (soy milk contains healthful fats). You can use the soybean, the chocolate, or vanilla flavor. Add honey instead of sugar or artificial sweeteners (one teaspoon). Each teaspoon of honey contains 15 calories as well as a high level of antioxidants and minerals. It is a more healthful sweetener than "toxic." (I'd rather drink my coffee bitter than with an artificial sweetener or processed sugar.)

You may add dried cardamom pods to taste (four to five seeds per cup). Cardamom dilates capillaries all over the body, including those in the brain and under the skin, and it can counteract the hypertensive effect of caffeinated coffee. It also increases memory.

Take one to two cups of water for each cup of coffee to counteract its dehydration effect. In my country, when you sit in a coffee shop, they bring you the small Turkish cup, bitter coffee or coffee with sugar, and a cup of water will be in the same tray.

If you drink the farmer's son's coffee instead of your usual cup of coffee, I believe that you will not lose a year of your life, and you might even add a year (if not more) to your life.

The farmer's son's coffee has no processed sugar or saturated fats and doesn't increase blood pressure; the soy milk has the plant phytoestrogens, which are an anticancer. The coffee amount is up to 400 mg per day (four cups) or 8 oz each.

Aboya Coffee (My Father's Coffee)

For all coffee makers, use fresh, ground, medium roasted coffee.

Cold water 8 oz	Ground coffee 1 tbsp	Cardamom pods 3 to 5 pods	Calcium-fortified soy milk, vanilla, or chocolate flavor 3 tbsp	Natural honey 1 tsp for overweight and diabetics (15 calories), 2 tsp for underweight

Add the cardamom and the ground coffee to 8 oz cold water.
Brew the coffee.
Fix your cup with the soy milk and honey.
Enjoy.

Beneficial Factors of Aboya Coffee

Cardamom	Vasodilator for the brain and small arterial vessels. It reduces blood pressure, which counteracts the vasoconstriction. Caffeine has a nice flavor and improves memory function.
Soy milk	It has no saturated fat. It has the good fats. It has the plant estrogen with its anticancer action, especially for the breast cancer. It improves cholesterol.
Natural honey	It has sugar (glucose and fructose, antioxidants, minerals, vitamins, and trace elements.) It does not leach the body of nutrients when used as a nutritious sweetener.

This coffee has less toxic chemicals and preserves health while giving the coffee benefits.

Comparison Between Aboya Coffee and Regular Coffee

Regular Coffee	Aboya coffee
Has caffeine; it increases the blood pressure by vasoconstriction of subcutaneous capillaries.	No or less blood pressure increase.
It has saturated fat.	Good fats, poly- and monounsaturated fats
It has processed sugar according to the book *Sugar Busters*. It is toxic. It leaches your body nutrients. NutraSweet when used is not better either.	It has the honey with all the nutrients needed to be used by the body.
It is usually not flavored.	Can be flavored.

Tea

It is made of leaves (the antioxidant, anticancer, and antibacterial factor).

Tea is one of the most popular beverages in China, Japan, and Britain. Green tea is the most healthful of all teas followed in order of highest benefit by white tea and then black tea. The caffeine content of green, black, and white tea varies, although all three varieties are antioxidants and exert antiviral, antibacterial, and antitumor effects. If we compare 8 oz cups of black, green, and white tea, we find that black tea contains 40 mg of caffeine, green tea contains 10 mg of caffeine (and the highest level of antioxidants), and white tea contains 5 mg of caffeine.

The antioxidants in tea are primarily polyphenols, which exert antiviral, antibacterial, and anticancer effects. For example, the anticancer effect of green tea occurs when the antioxidants in the tea cause quickly dividing cancer cells to stick together, which prevent them to metastasize. Without affecting healthy cells, the antioxidants in tea inhibit the growth of new blood vessels needed to supply tumor cells; this disrupts the growth of the tumor.

Drinking one cup of green tea every day will lower high blood pressure up to 7 percent (as shown in research done in China), but coffee temporarily increases blood pressure.

Green tea, which contains epigallocatechin gallate (EGCG), benefits people with an autoimmune disease in which the body identifies its own cells (perhaps in the intestine or colon) as being foreign and produces antibodies to attack those cells. EGCG suppresses the inflammation that occurs when the body attacks its own cells, and it also inhibits the activity of the antigens that trigger an autoimmune response.

White tea and green tea are the teas most effective against cancers of the prostate or ovary.

Tea inhibits the bacteria that flourish in gums afflicted with gingivitis.

Green tea benefits people with some autoimmune diseases (illnesses in which the body misidentifies its own cells as foreign invading organisms and produces antibodies to attack its own healthy cells) such as psoriasis. Green tea contains the chemical epigallocatechin gallate (EGCG), which suppresses inflammation and inhibits the activity of antigens that triggers an autoimmune response.

Both white and green teas exert a protective effect against cancer, especially cancer of the prostate or ovary.

If they are used three times daily for a few months as an oral rinse, those types of tea contribute to good oral health by preventing gingivitis, inhibiting the action of oral bacteria, and reducing dental plaque.

Although caffeine can cause dehydration, increase urination, improve alertness and concentration and make you feel better, tea (especially green tea) behaves like a nutrient.

Some caffeine (but only a small amount) is found in green or white tea.

You can drink from one to six eight-ounce cups of tea each day; however, limit your caffeine intake from tea to 400 mg or less per day.

Don't drink tea on an empty stomach; doing so can increase gastric acid, cause heartburn, increase your heart rate, and produce nausea. Remember that tea has the following effects:

- It is beneficial for cells and functions as a nutrient.
- It is an anti-free radical agent.

- It is an anticancer agent.
- Reduces the level of bad cholesterol.
- Reduces blood pressure.
- Inhibits the bacteria that flourish in gums afflicted with gingivitis.
- Reduces oral plaque if used for several months as a daily oral three-minute rinse.

When compared with coffee, tea contains less caffeine (a substance that can cause dehydration, increase urination and alertness, and improve mood and concentration).

Tea, especially green tea, exerts antioxidant, anti-inflammatory, antiviral, antibacterial, and anticarcinogenic (anticancer) effects.

Coffee, however, improves vision, improves concentration and cognition, improves memory, is addictive, can increase blood pressure, and stimulates brain function.

If you like coffee and tea, it's a good idea to consume both each day, but to consume more tea than coffee, remember these facts about coffee and tea:

- Drink coffee in the morning after breakfast to reduce the likelihood of gastric reflux and to increase alertness.
- Drink tea at lunch because then you are more awake.
- Drink coffee at the end of the day to relieve fatigue.
- A second and third cup of green tea, which is an antioxidant, is okay; it increases alertness. Add some sage or rosemary to green tea to improve memory.
- If you have a long drive ahead, drink a cup of coffee to increase alertness, but remember that an 8 oz cup of coffee contains 100 mg of caffeine.

- Tea with a little sugar or no sugar can increase satiety and energy, and the ECGC that it contains can help with weight loss.
- Antioxidants like tea decrease the levels of bad cholesterol and triglyceride.

The Farmer's Son's Tea

Green tea plus sage if you do not want to start forgetting things. If you add rosemary to sage, it gives a stronger memory factor.

Green tea plus anise and chamomile. If you can't sleep or you're nervous, it is nerve soothing.

Regular tea, if you like it, plus three to four cardamom seeds to keep blood pressure stable and improve memory.

In my case, I add to green tea multiple types of tea, cinnamon, hibiscus, chamomile, and anise; it tastes good. Total caffeine is low; and benefits for the nerve (soothing), memory, and antioxidants are high. Don't take any type of NutraSweet or Sweet'n Low; it will reduce the tea's effect on the memory and brain. I add one spoonful of natural honey or 15 calories to my tea. I'd rather use one teaspoonful of sugar (15 calories) than taking any NutraSweet.

A Sweet Addiction: High-fructose Corn Syrup

The 150 to 160 lb of sugar that most Americans consume annually consists primarily of sucrose and fructose. Sweeter than sugar, fructose is found naturally in fruits; it accounts for 7 percent of the weight of cherries, pears, bananas, and grapes and for half that amount in strawberries, oranges, and grapefruit. The intestinal absorption of fructose requires no enzymatic action because fructose is a simple sugar, and fructose intolerance is a rare condition.

Processed fructose was first made available in the United States around 1980 via the icy fermentation of cornstarch, a method devised in Japan. In 1970, the sugar beet became the primary source of fructose. Fructose from sugar beets requires less insulin for its conversion to energy. Beet sugar increases blood clotting, blood pressure, and the levels of uric acid and bad cholesterol. It contributes to obesity, decreases the levels of good cholesterol and triglyceride, worsens gout and diabetes, and may cause insulin resistance, so fructose made from sugar beets should be consumed in minimal amounts. However, the absorption of sugar beet requires glucose. Without which, it is transported to the colon and produces intestinal gas. For that reason, the fructose in beet sugar is combined with glucose to form high-fructose corn syrup (HFCS), which consists of 55 percent fructose and 45 percent glucose.

HFCS is the food additive that has most contributed to the obesity of Americans over the last two decades. A sweetener that contains 60 calories per tablespoon, HFCS is added to an alarming number of foods sold in America. It mixes easily into other foods, is relatively inexpensive, has a long shelf life, and inhibits the hormone that produces satiety (a feeling of having eaten enough). However, the fructose in fruits (which also contain abundant vitamins, antioxidants, and minerals) and starches is not a processed substance. Processed fructose is really a refined sugar, and although it can be consumed in small amounts, its overconsumption causes the problems associated with a diet high in processed sugar. A high-fructose diet causes a high level of blood sugar and can produce intestinal cramps, loose stools, and bloating. Bacteria, which thrive on fructose, can increase intestinal gas.

Research suggests that the excessive consumption of HFCS may increase the United States incidence of nonalcoholic fatty liver disease (as well as that of diabetes and obesity) and may also contribute to human aging and atherosclerosis. A diet high in HFCS is linked with the development of vascular, renal, and ocular disease in diabetic patients and may be the primary cause of chronic diarrhea and other disorders of bowel function. However, the amount of fructose that occurs naturally in fruits and vegetables is unlikely to exert a harmful effect on health, and fruits and vegetables are sources of essential vitamins and minerals.

A diet high in HFCS can also lead to the development of the metabolic syndrome (a collection of risk factors for both cardiovascular disease and insulin resistance) and is linked with various neurodegenerative diseases. HFCS increases the level of uric acid in blood and urine, causes gout, and increases the level of inorganic phosphate, which in turn depletes energy. It stimulates the liver and produces high levels of fatty acids and triglyceride. Consuming a small amount of HFCS daily is not harmful, but a twelve-ounce soft drink contains thirteen teaspoons of that sweetener, and some soft drinks can now be purchased in thirty-six-ounce servings! In fact, Americans now drink twice the amount of soda (up to fifty-six gallons per year) than the amount they consumed in 1990. Our high consumption of sugar has had another unfortunate effect. Since 1980, which marked the beginning of the increase in fructose consumption, milk consumption in the United States has decreased by 50 percent.

In healthy people, high levels of leptin (a hormone produced by fat cells) and insulin tell the brain that the body has had enough food and that no more eating is necessary. HFCS, however, blocks that message, so appetite is not satisfied and eating continues. For that reason, I consider fructose to be an addictive food; it does not induce satiety. In addition, HFCS does not suppress the hormone ghrelin, which stimulates appetite.

Some experts suggest that the United States intake of HFCS may now exceed that of sucrose. However, other sweeteners can be used instead of refined sugar or HFCS. Molasses, which is derived from beer, has about the same calorie count as that of corn syrup. One tablespoon of granulated sugar contains about 80 calories, and one tablespoon of honey has about 60 calories. I suggest substituting one teaspoon of honey, which contains 15 calories and trace amounts of some nutrients for refined sugar.

Honey

Unlike refined sugar, honey is not toxic. It is the best source of calories consumed before and after exercise. Honey contains polyphenols and other antioxidants, minerals, and vitamins. The darker the honey, the more antioxidants it contains.

One tablespoon (21 g) of honey contains the following:

- 0.5 g of protein
- 15 to 17 g of carbohydrates half as sucrose and glucose and the other half is fructose
- 60 to 70 calories (half the calories in one tablespoon of olive oil)

Here are some differences between table (refined) sugar and honey:

- Table sugar decreases insulin sensitivity; honey does not do so.
- Table sugar decreases immunity; honey improves immunity.
- Table sugar leaches nutrients from the body; honey contains these nutrients.

- Sugar is carcinogenic; honey does not cause cancer.
- Sugar decreases calcium absorption and weakens bones; honey increases calcium absorption and strengthens bones.
- Honey exerts antiallergic and antioxidant effects and contains same calories per teaspoon as table sugar.
- The prophet Mohammed suggested honey; it has a flavor, is full of nutrients, and is antibacterial.
- It's a natural healer for burns and wounds because it has low water content; it kills bacteria by dehydrating the wound.
- It forms peroxide when it sucks the water from the wound, giving more antibacterial effect.
- The action of its antioxidants, back home they cover superficial burns with it; it reduces the pain in minutes.
- Also it increases immunity and energy when taken by mouth.

Honey, the bee pollen honey, is of different color and sources according to the type of flower nectar. The bee honey contains millions of these pollens and the bee digestive enzymes.

Bee pollen honey, which contains nutrients and trace elements, is very nutritious. It is a powerful antioxidant that is used in food supplements and skin creams.

Royal Jelly

Royal jelly, a substance that is produced by the salivary glands of worker bees, is a life extender. It contains a high level of flavonoids with the most potent anti-free radical agents. Royal jelly extends the life of the queen bee. It contains minerals, proteins, vitamins (mostly vitamin B), amino acids, and fatty acids. One tablespoon of royal jelly contains five hundred times more flavonoids than a medium-size orange and two hundred times more antioxidants than a medium-size apple. In addition, royal jelly exerts antibacterial, antifungal, and antiviral effects. Eat in small amounts.

Food Dressings

Catsup

Catsup is a staple in the American diet. Made from ripe tomatoes and flavored with vinegar, salt, sugar, various blends of spices, and sometimes added vegetables, it is a nutritious low-calorie complement to many foods. A small combination pack of two types of catsup (both of which are low in protein and fat) that is particularly handy contains the following:

- Low-salt tomato catsup, which is good for people with high blood pressure or diabetes. Each tablespoon of this catsup contains 30 calories and 275 milligrams of sodium (high content).
- Hot brown salsa catsup, which contains a half calorie per gram and 150 mg of sodium.
- Chili catsup, which contains capsaicin and hot pepper, is also available; it is usually low in calories. Catsup may also contain sugar, grape juice, pepper, celery, cider vinegar, chili peppers, and various spices.

Raw Hot Chili Peppers

Raw chili peppers contain low calories; water; fiber; carbohydrates; vitamins A, C (110 mg), and K; minerals such as calcium, iron, potassium, and magnesium, vitamin B6 and C.

Don't eat too much of it to avoid possibility of stomach cancer.

Chili

Chili contains the following:

- Tomato (a source of lycopene and vitamin C)
- Onion (a source of chromium and quercetin)
- Beans (which contain vitamins and minerals)
- Antioxidants
- Capsaicin (which provides the hot spicy taste, increases oxygen consumption, and causes a feeling of warmth)

Chili is a versatile dish with varied ingredients, is low in calories and fat, and contains vitamins and minerals. Some brands of canned chili are high in salt, so be sure to read the label if you must limit your salt intake.

Ranch Dressing

Ranch dressing is high in sodium and is not good in hypertension.

Ranch dressing adds flavor to salads and is often used as a dipping sauce. It is high in sodium, fat, and calories and usually contains buttermilk, sour cream, white wine vinegar, mayonnaise, onion, garlic, fresh olives, and salt.

One tablespoon of ranch dressing contains 75 calories, 9 grams of fat, and 122 mg of sodium as well as calcium, potassium, magnesium, and vitamin A. Ranch dressing is good for active young people but not for those with diabetes or a high cholesterol level. If you love ranch dressing, choose the light or low-fat type, which is low in calories and provides all the benefits of regular ranch dressing but only half the fat. However, the light version is high in sodium (one tablespoon can contain as much as 325 mg of sodium), so although it is a good choice for dieters, it should not be consumed by people with kidney or heart disease or high blood pressure.

Blue Cheese Dressing

Avoid this if you have high cholesterol, kidney disease, and heart disease. It has high sodium; avoid in hypertension cases.

Blue cheese dressing is added to salads and is used as a dipping sauce. It is high in calories, saturated fat, and sodium, and it usually contains sugar, vinegar, garlic, salt, mayonnaise, and sour cream.

One ounce of blue cheese dressing contains 100 calories, 8 g of fat (total), 5 g of saturated fat (very high), and 400 mg of sodium.

Ginger: The Motion Sickness Factor

The root of the ginger plant provides a flavorful spice that is used in cooking. Ginger root is also eaten in pickled form, in tea, or in hot soup. The oil in ginger provides this spice with its characteristic taste. Ginger relieves motion sickness and nausea (even that caused by chemotherapy) by blocking a product of oxidation that stimulates the cells of the stomach and causes vomiting. To prevent airsickness or motion sickness, you can take two 500 mg tablets of ginger before you fly or begin a drive. Considered the spice most beneficial after garlic, ginger have these benefits:

- Relieves spasms, menstrual cramps, hot flashes, flatulence, morning sickness, and fever.
- It is a vasodilator that reduces high blood pressure.;

- It improves digestion and appetite.
- It is a blood thinner (so do not eat ginger if you take warfarin [Coumadin]).
- It improves appetite.

Remember that consuming a large amount of ginger can cause an upset stomach.

Horseradish

Horseradish is a popular pungent seasoning that is a diuretic, relieves asthma, exerts an anti-inflammatory effect that clears the sinuses, and improves digestion and appetite.

Mustard: A Gastric and Pancreatic Juice Stimulant

Mustard is a spice known for its characteristic yellow color and its hot, pungent flavor. This flavorful spice is made from ground mustard seeds. One tablespoon of mustard contains the following:

- 50 calories
- A minimal amount of fat
- No cholesterol or saturated fat
- Some calcium
- A minimal amount of sodium
- Vitamin C
- Selenium
- Some fiber
- Manganese
- Magnesium

Mustard

This spice is nutrient rich, is good for your health, exerts an anti-inflammatory effect, helps to relieve arthritis, stimulates gastric and pancreatic secretions, and is often eaten with hot dogs.

Sumac: An Aid to Digestion

The spice sumac is made from the crushed dried berries of a wild bush that grows in Mediterranean countries such as Lebanon. Sumac powder is purple. This flavorful spice

- improves digestion;
- is used in Middle Eastern cuisine (especially shish kabobs);
- is high in vitamin C;
- heals lesions caused by poison ivy;
- can be made into a tea that relieves diarrhea;
- was once used to treat diabetes and tuberculosis; and
- contains iodine, several acids (egg, tartaric acid, tannic acid), and many minerals, all of which are good for the stomach

Vanilla: The Manganese Factor

Vanilla, which is one of the most frequently used spices, is obtained from the greenish yellow cup of the vanilla plant. Vanilla is used in desserts, ice cream, and candy. One tablespoon (15 g) of vanilla, which contains 30 calories and no fat, is low in sodium and high in potassium.

One cup or 200 grams contain manganese or 23 percent DV; riboflavin 13 percent, and 8 percent DV of each carbohydrate all as sugar form, magnesium, potassium, and copper.

CHAPTER 6

Antioxidants

It is important to decrease the effects of free radicals, free radicals are the aging factor. it can cause eye diseases and disorders of the lens and retina, the formation of blood clots, and chronic degenerative conditions such as arthritis, heart disease, or Parkinson's disease. Free radicals accelerate aging, shorten the life of nerve cells, and narrow the diameter of blood vessels.

To prevent the damage caused by free radicals, increase your consumption of antioxidants (which are free radical scavengers) by consuming nutrients like those listed below.

- Phytochemicals from fruits and vegetables.
- Carotenoid, beta-carotene, lycopene, and lutein, which are found in citrus fruits, carrots, and sweet potatoes.
- Polyphenols, which protect against the big four—cancer, diabetes, heart failure, and strokes—and are found in tea (the highest), red wine, cocoa, and vegetables such as cabbage (Research done by Dr. N. Holenberg at Harvard Medical School.) Polyphenols, which are found in oregano and rosemary and are good for brain function and memory

- Flavonoids, such as anthocyanin, and quercetin, which reduce the levels of bad cholesterol and the likelihood of blood clotting and protect against cancer. Flavonoids are found in red grapes, tea (again), berries, fruits, vegetables such as green beans and onions, and red wine.
- Flavones, which reduce the risk of breast cancer and prostate cancer. These are found in citrus, tea (again), and wine.
- Genistein, which is a phytoestrogen, and is found in olive oil, soybeans, soy milk, and tofu. It is an anticancer, reduces osteoporosis, and reduces hot flashes and heart disease.
- Caffeic acid, which are found in coffee berries and other fruits, is a carcinogenic inhibitor and protects the skin from UV rays.
- Resveratrol, which is important to heart function and are found in grapes and blueberries.
- Sulfides (like those found in garlic and onion), which exert antibacterial and ant carcinogenic effects. They are especially protective against colon cancer.
- Lutein and zeaxanthin, which occur in egg yolks and corn, is beta-carotenoids, protects the eye from free radicals secondary to UV light.
- Methionine, which is found in meat.
- Coenzyme Q10, which is in meat, whole grains, and fish and inhibits the growth of cancer cells. This enzyme is more effective if it is taken with vitamin C.
- Zinc, which is found in meat, grains, beans, and seeds, is good for eye health.
- Vitamin E, which occurs in nuts, seeds, and grains and recycles or recharges and already used other vitamins and antioxidants, such as vitamin C and coenzyme Q10.

- Vitamin C, which exerts an anticancer effect and recycles or recharges vitamin E. Citrus fruits are high in vitamin C.
- Alpha-lipoic acid, which is found in liver and kidney meats, spinach and broccoli and potato, reduces deficiency of vitamin C and E and decreases mitochondria decay.
- Selenium and copper as part of enzymes, which are essential for antioxidants to work; Brazil nuts is a good source.

Fruits High in Antioxidants

Blackberries and blueberries are among the foods with the highest levels of antioxidants, but those fruits are high in calories. Other foods that have a low or moderate calorie count and are also high in antioxidants include the following:

- Strawberries (a moderate calorie count)
- Garlic (minimal calories)
- Brussels sprouts, broccoli, and fresh red peppers (low in calories)
- Black or red grapes (a moderate calorie count). The French have a lower incidence of heart attack than do Americans, perhaps in part because they consume a diet high in red and black grapes. Those types of grapes, like wine, has the resveratrol, which improves heart function and circulation. However, for many people, eating grapes can be safer than drinking an alcoholic beverage as wine.
- Red apples, a medium apple, with moderate calories (has the highest in all other apples)
- Beans, seeds, and nuts, which are high in antioxidants and in calories. Red beans is the highest.
- Thyme, pomegranate, and honey, which are higher in antioxidants than are the foods listed above.

Most of us probably consume our highest levels of antioxidants in coffee, tea (especially green tea), and beans not because those foods are highest in antioxidants but because they are consumed often and in large amounts.

Antioxidants, which may help to reduce the risk for cancer and age-related macular degeneration. According to the United States Department of Agriculture (USDA), high levels of antioxidants are found in the foods listed below.

Antioxidant Values

Antioxidant values are measured by their total antioxidant capacity (TAC) or their oxygen radical absorption capacity (ORAC). Below is the list of foods high in antioxidants. The quantity of each food listed is one serving, which equals to one cup (unless otherwise specified) or a portion weighing 130 to 160 grams. The values are expressed in ORAC units, and the higher the value the better.

Fruits

Blueberries: 10,000 to 13,000
Cranberries: 9,000
Blackberries: 8,000
Apple (1 red, medium size): 6,000 ORAC units
Strawberries: 6,000
Raspberries: 6,000
Avocado: 5,000
Cherries: 5,000
Plum (1 medium size): 4,000
Orange (1 medium size): 3,000

Pear (1 medium size): 3,000
½ cup of figs: 3,000
Red grapes: 2,000
Grapefruit (half): 2,000
Peach: 2,000
Banana (1 medium size): 1,000
Broccoli: 600
Cantaloupe: 600

Beans and Vegetables (One Cup)

Red beans (dried) 13,500. The highest in all fruits and vegetables.
Pinto beans: 11,000
Black beans: 4,000
Navy beans: 3,000

Vegetables

Artichoke (1 medium size): 8,000
Eggplant: 1,000
Corn (uncooked): 600
Carrot (raw): 700, cooked: 200
Baby carrots: 300

Here are the ORAC values for one ounce of the following nuts and dried fruits:

Pecans: 5,000
Walnuts: 4,000
Pistachios: 2,000

Peanuts: 1,000
Raisins: 1,000
Dates: 1,000

Here are the ORAC values for one ounce of the following spices:

Thyme, 1 oz Is 30,000 ORAC, the highest in all spices
Cloves (ground): 3,000
Cinnamon: 2,500
Curry powder: 500
Ginger: 200
Mustard powder: 200
Garlic: 200
Pepper (ground): 200

Remember the following:

Beans are good foods, has high protein, fiber, and antioxidants, but they have a high glycemic load; so eat a quarter cup, but a cup is good if you just finished running a marathoner or is underweight.

Nuts are also good. They have the good fats, but they are high in calories. Consuming antioxidants in spices is a good idea because a small amount of some spices has a high antioxidant value. The cheapest and the lowest in calories is thyme.

A 140 g red apple has 5,000 ORAC.
A 150 g thyme gives 150,000 ORAC.
So if you eat 5 g or one teaspoonful thyme powder, you have
    ORAC as much as an apple.

Royal Jelly

It has very high content of antioxidants.

Royal jelly has the highest antioxidant ORAC from all foods; one g has 1100 ORAC.

So the following foods has the highest antioxidant content:

Royal jelly
Oregano (thyme, or zaater)
Black raspberry
Pomegranate
Blueberry

Note: Zaatar (thyme) has the least calorie content.

CHAPTER 7

Vitamins, Omega-3, and Minerals

Omega-3.

The term *omega-3* refers to three essential fatty acids (ALA,EPA, AND DHA) supplied in foods or as a supplement.

Omega-6 (which contains linolenic fatty acid found in sunflower, corn, and soybean oils and arachidonic acid found in the egg yolk and meat) and omega-3 compete on the same enzymes; that's why we want you to take the more beneficial one. We suggest the ratio of omega-3 to omega-6 to be one to three and even later one to one.

Omega-3 is found in cold-water fish, such as salmon, sardines, and tuna; in nuts such as walnuts and in flaxseed. It is given as capsules of 1,000 mg, one to three times per day.

Adverse Effects of Omega-3

In people with diabetes or heart disease, omega-3 can increase the levels of blood sugar and/or bad cholesterol, but that effect can be counteracted by vitamins E or C (I suggest taking Ester-C because it is not fat soluble, and it is effective for many hours). Omega-3 should be spaced four hours with the cholesterol-lowering medication (pravastatin and simvastatin or with immunosuppressive drug such as cyclosporine) and given to transplant patients.

Patients taking omega-3 and coenzyme Q10 is okay, but taking omega-3 plus vitamin A or niacin is not recommended.

Niacin (Vitamin B3)

Niacin is the factor to increase good cholesterol and the best in lowering high triglycerides.

Here are some facts to remember about niacin (vitamin B3):

- The daily value of niacin for an adult is 33 mg.
- A deficiency in niacin causes pellagra, which is characterized by cracked, scaly, and discolored skin.
- Niacin is essential for the repair of deoxyribonucleic acid (DNA) and is needed (in addition to fatty acids) to build every cell in the body.
- It is essential for conversion of carbohydrate to glucose to be used by the cells for energy.
- Like the hormones called *steroids,* niacin is important for insulin function.
- Niacin prevents the development of diabetes, eye diseases such as glaucoma, Alzheimer's disease, and low thyroid function.

Adverse Effects of Niacin

This important vitamin, however, does cause some adverse effects. It causes annoying flushing of the face and neck and can produce low blood pressure and dizziness. Nicotinic acid has the same effect, although the recommended daily value of niacin is up to 2 g daily and that of nicotinic acid is 100 to 200 mg per day. A formulation of niacin that does not cause flushing is available over the counter, but that product has not been approved by the US Food and Drug Administration (FDA).

Remember these facts about niacin:

- It reduces the level of total cholesterol.
- It increases the level of good cholesterol. (Also, eating walnuts, exercising, consuming olive oil, or taking a vacation can also increase the level of good cholesterol).
- It is good for memory, as are curry, sage, and rosemary tea.
- It is found in meat, peanuts, and seafood.
- It can be prescribed in therapeutic doses to treat a high level of triglyceride, which is a type of fat. When the level of triglyceride in the bloodstream is too high (hypertriglyceridemia), as it often is in people with diabetes or a genetic predisposition to the development of hypertriglyceridemia, the blood becomes whitish yellow. In healthy people, the level of triglyceride is usually less than 150 mg/dl, but in those with hypertriglyceridemia, that level may be thousands of milligrams per deciliter. Hypertriglyceridemia can cause microvascular diseases. However, many medications used to treat. Clofibrate and statins have less effect on the triglyceride level than niacin does. However, the least expensive and most effective agent for lowering a too-high triglyceride level is omega-3 in a

dosage ranging from 1 g twice daily to 4 g daily, plus a diet that has a low glycemic load, low in saturated fat and high in antioxidants and carbohydrates, and includes a vitamin B complex supplement containing niacin and nicotinic acid in tolerable amounts. If the results of your blood test reveal that your level of triglyceride is high, watch for the signs of diabetes.

- A high intake of niacin can increase the level of homocysteine, so take 400 mcg of folic acid (to reduce homocysteine) with your niacin supplement.
- Do not take niacin with a statin.
- Do not take niacin with a calcium channel blocker such as amlodipine besylate (Norvasc).
- Do not take niacin if you have liver disease.
- Be sure that you have your doctor's approval before you take niacin, especially if you are also taking any medication.
- The RDA for niacin is 20 mg per day. The RDA is usually the lowest amount of a nutrient that is needed to prevent a disease; it is not the amount recommended for the treatment of a disease.

Food sources of niacin include

- 4 oz of chicken breast, which provides 75 percent of the daily value of niacin;
- 4 oz of tuna, salmon, or sardines, which provides 50 percent of the daily value of niacin;
- 3 oz or 5 mg of lamb, beef, or turkey;
- 2 tbsp or 4 mg of peanuts;

- 5 oz of green beans, which provides 25 percent of the daily value of niacin; and
- 5 oz of raw mushrooms, which provides 25 percent of the daily value of niacin.

Vitamin E: Antioxidant which can cross the cell wall) and a Blood Thinner

Vitamin E (alpha-tocopherol) reduces the risk for stroke. It is not formed in the body as are the essential fatty acids and amino acids. Remember the following about vitamin E, which is one of the most beneficial vitamins:

- Slows aging
- Prevents degenerative conditions
- Thins the blood and thus prevents blood clots
- Improves the symptoms of arthritis
- Bolsters immunity
- Protects against Alzheimer's disease
- Eliminates acne
- Protects against cataracts
- Improves insulin function and stimulates insulin secretion (good for diabetics)
- Decreases the levels of bad cholesterol
- Protects against stroke if taken with one baby aspirin each day. In some people, however, taking one baby aspirin daily causes excess gastric acid or esophageal reflux. Vitamin E can replace aspirin for those who cannot take that aspirin. in this case 600 to 800 mcg is given per day
- Is good for people with epilepsy

- Has a recommended dosage of 400 mcg, with a baby aspirin, and/or 400 mcg twice a day if aspirin is contraindicated
- Is a good antioxidant at the cellular level
- Is found in peanuts, liver, sesame seeds, tomatoes, red peppers, cheese.
- Should not be taken in a dose of more than 1,000 mcg daily unless that amount is prescribed by a doctor.
- Can be taken with vitamin A to increase its anti-platelet effect.
- Can be taken with vitamin C to recharge vitamin E when oxidized. Protegra (OTC medicine) is a good source.

Just remember that

- vitamin E thins the blood,
- vitamin C improves vascular health and protects against infections,
- folic acid improves heart health.

Just to be on the safe side, do not take too much of *anything*. Taking too many vitamins or too large a dose of a specific vitamin may not be the best thing for your health, so please consume those nutrients in a moderate amount.

Biotin: Retina Energy Factor

Biotin is good to create energy to the nerve cells. For that reason, biotin is good for the retinal nerves and relieves postexercise muscle pain. A deficiency in biotin can cause ataxia, a lack of muscle coordination that results in poor muscle tone.

Vitamin K: The Clotting Factor

This vitamin heals bruises. It also

- improves the health of the capillaries and prevents their rupture;
- strengthens the collagen layer (which makes the capillaries stronger) when taken with vitamin C; and
- protects against osteoporosis.

It is found in sunflowers, liver, fruits, vegetables, and soybeans.

However, in my opinion, you should not take vitamin K tablets without your doctor's approval.

Vitamin B6: For Vomiting in the First Trimester of Pregnancy

Vitamin B6 (pyridoxine) is needed for the formation of DNA and ribonucleic acid (RNA), which carry genetic information and ensure normal cell function, as well as for the metabolism of certain hormones and saccharin. Vitamin B6 is important for hydrochloric acid secretion in the stomach and the absorption of carbohydrates and protein.

It has the following benefits:

- Improves immunity
- Facilitates wound healing
- Protects against atherosclerosis

- Protects against asthma
- Is recommended in a daily dosage of 2 mg daily (the RDA), but taking 10 mg per day is OK as directed by your doctor for special indications
- Is beneficial for pregnant women who experience nausea and vomiting during the first three months of pregnancy (however, pregnant women should consult their doctor before they take any medication or supplement)
- Exerts an antiviral and antibacterial effect
- Enhances antibody protection

Folic Acid: The Antihomocysteine Factor (A Separate Inflammatory Factor)

Folic acid is another essential vitamin. In the United States today, 30 percent of our adult population and 11 percent of all population consume a low level of folic acid. The RDA of folic acid is 400 mcg. However, the foods and beverages that you consume each day usually supply about 150 mcg of folic acid daily, so you may need to supplement your intake of this vitamin. People older than forty years who have a health problem such as celiac disease, which results in malabsorption or multiple negative health factors require 1 mg of folic acid daily. If you have a specific health problem, your doctor may prescribe a larger dose of folic acid.

This vitamin has the following benefits:

- This is good for red blood cells.
- It is beneficial for people with anemia.

- It attaches to homocysteine and prevents it from attaching to particles of bad cholesterol that can injure inner blood vessel walls and clog arteries.
- It improves appetite.

It is present in soybeans, wheat grains, beans, liver, meat, and asparagus.

Vitamin B12: The Antihallucination Factor

Vitamin B12, which is a very important vitamin, is sometimes referred to as the *antihallucination factor*. It protects against physical and mental illnesses in the elderly. Vitamin B12 can be consumed in foods, taken orally as a tablet or a sublingual troche, or injected.

It improves mental activity, prevents pernicious anemia, benefits nervous system function, nourishes the covering of the nerves (especially those in the brain), helps relieve irritability and hallucinations in those aged sixty-five or seventy years when administered by injection.

Vitamin C: A Major Antioxidant,

Vitamin C is often called the *capillary health factor*. A deficiency of that vitamin leads to acute scurvy, which afflicted many sailors in years past. Scurvy is characterized by poor healing, loose teeth, fragile blood vessels, subcutaneous bleeding, mild anemia, and possible gastric bleeding.

Remember that vitamin C

- is one of the most frequently ingested vitamins,
- is nontoxic even in high doses,
- exerts an anti-inflammatory effect,
- is good for those with rheumatoid arthritis,
- benefits people with chronic obstructive lung disease,
- works like a beta-blocker to reduce the heart rate,
- reduces the levels of bad cholesterol,
- reduces the plaques that blocks arteries.
- reduces the risk for recurrent heart attacks in those older than sixty-five years.
- strengthens the walls of small blood vessels and capillaries by increasing their collagen content, which renders them less susceptible to injury and subsequent leakage,
- exerts an antioxidant effect, and
- benefits blood synthesis.

If you have a viral or bacterial infection, you may need to double the amount of vitamin C that you consume daily. I suggest that you take 500 mg of vitamin C twice daily if you have no health conditions like those listed below or 2 g per day if you do have any of those health challenges.

- Diabetes
- High blood pressure
- Obesity
- Smoking
- High levels of bad cholesterol

People who cannot take aspirin to thin their blood can take 400 mcg of vitamin E plus 500 mg of vitamin C once or twice daily. However, those with kidney stones should not supplement their diet with vitamin C, which produces oxalic acid, a substance that increases the incidence of kidney stone formation.

Vitamin C is found in oranges, cantaloupes, watermelon, tomatoes, lemonade, bananas, strawberries, and most fruits and vegetables.

Multivitamins

I would like to say something about vitamins A, E, and C as well as omega-3 fatty acids. If taken regularly or in high doses, those nutrients can affect platelet function because they thin the blood as aspirin does. Please inform your doctor about all the prescribed and over-the-counter medications and supplements that you take. Please stop taking vitamins A, E, and C and omega-3 fatty acids four days before any surgery that you must undergo, especially operations on structures that cannot expand to accommodate the volume of blood from any procedure-related bleeding like eye and brain surgeries.

Subcutaneous bleeding can stretch the skin, which can accommodate about 30 ml of blood. Although subcutaneous bleeding is not serious even if an infection develops at the site of swelling, bleeding involving even a few milliliters of blood in the eye can temporarily or even permanently damage vision. Often bleeding from a small aneurysm in the eye cannot be stopped, but bleeding caused by aspirin or vitamin C intake usually can be halted. You must not take those medications until two days after surgery at which time any beneficial postsurgical blood clots are firmly in place. Notice that I said *medications* and not *vitamins*. It is important to stop taking vitamins and other supplements a few days before any operation because excessive bleeding might occur. Such bleeding can often be managed in a hospital but not in an office setting.

Vitamin D: The Bone Factor

Vitamin D, which is found in dairy products, salmon, and herring, is called the bone-building factor. It is essential for the absorption of calcium and the formation of new bone. Vitamin D and calcium (both of which are essential to bone development and can prevent, stop, or even improve osteoporosis) should be consumed together. Exposure to the sun can increase your level of vitamin D.

Vitamin Toxicity

The vitamins mentioned in this chapter are beneficial in recommended daily doses, but if taken in excess, they can be toxic. Vitamins A, D, and B6 are most likely to produce a toxic reaction. With the exception of vitamin B6, the B vitamins are the least toxic. Vitamin D can be toxic if a dose that is even slightly higher than the recommended daily requirement (about 400 mcg per day) is taken every day. Now let's examine the effects that the overconsumption of essential vitamins can cause.

Vitamin A

Do not take more than 5,000 IU of vitamin A daily or you can experience

- dry, yellow, scaly skin;
- blurred vision;
- dizziness;
- vomiting;
- joint pain;
- eye irritation;
- a high level of calcium in the bloodstream;
- a toxic reaction that affects the brain, if vitamin A is taken in high doses.

Remember the following:

- Pregnant and lactating women should take vitamin A only under medical supervision.
- Do not take beta-carotene if you have low thyroid function because then your body cannot convert beta-carotene into vitamin A.
- Do not administer high doses of vitamin A to children.

Vitamin D

Remember that the usual dose of vitamin D is 400 mcg a day. A doctor should decide the dose in pregnant women; if you take 1,000 mcg of vitamin D daily for about two months, you will experience a toxic reaction, such as hypocalcaemia with joint and limb pain, a metallic taste, stomach upset or pain, nausea, loss of appetite, constipation, and diarrhea.

Vitamin E

Signs of vitamin E toxicity include **double vision** (remember this one), headache, fatigue, and diarrhea.

Vitamin C Toxicity (Rare)

This beneficial vitamin can be toxic if consumed in excess.

Remember the following:

- Taking large amounts of vitamin C will cause a high level of oxalic acid or its salt, oxalate, both of which can cause kidney stones and gallbladder stones, especially if you also eat dark chocolate or spinach, which increases the amount of oxalate in the bloodstream.
- You have to take 15,000 mg or more of vitamin C to experience stomach distension and discomfort and/or diarrhea.
- To increase the absorption of calcium, take it with vitamin C.
- Vitamin C increases the effects of the blood-thinning medication warfarin.

Niacin

Niacin, which is also called *nicotinic acid,* can cause

- flushing, which is usually temporary and can be relieved by taking aspirin before a dose of niacin,
- hypotension,
- a sensation of warmth that is caused by the dilatation of the veins under the skin, dilatation of small arterial vessels, and a feeling mimicking that caused by low blood pressure.

Vitamin B1

- I have seen vitamin B1 in doses of up to 300 mg per tablet (a too-high dose) sold over the counter and without dosing recommendations. In years past, we administered 100 mg of intramuscular vitamin B1 to eliminate (for about eight hours) delirium tremens caused by alcohol withdrawal. I suggest taking 100 mg of vitamin B1 orally each day or 100 mg every two days. An excess of vitamin B1 usually affects the nerves, so you may experience a loss of sensation in your legs, weakness in the dorsiflexion of your foot and while you are extending your hands, burning feet, autonomic system neuropathy, which produces a feeling like that caused by low blood pressure, disorders of the urinary bladder, and encephalopathy (a brain condition).

Vitamin B6

This vitamin causes nerve damage when taken in high doses.

Folic Acid

Folic acid has little toxicity. Most over-the-counter vitamins provide a daily dose of 1 mg or less of folic acid, which is acceptable. Some experts suggest that 400 mcg of folic acid daily is sufficient unless you have a specific disease and your doctor directs you to increase that dosage.

Coenzyme Q10

Coenzyme Q10 (Diabetics, those with heart disease, muscular disease, or those over fifty, you need CoQ10.)

Coenzyme Q10, which is a "five-star supplement," improves systolic and essential hypertension and fuels cells called *mitochondria*, which produce energy. Of the ten coenzymes that have been identified, only coenzyme Q10 is found in the human body.

This coenzyme has the following facts:

- Increases the oxygen supply to the tissues.
- Improves circulation.
- Increases energy.
- Exerts antioxidant and antiaging effects.
- Improves immunity.
- Acts as an antihistamine to help relieve the symptoms of asthma and autoimmune diseases.
- Benefits those with a brain disease or a psychiatric disorder.
- In young people, it is found in a high concentration in the heart, muscles, liver, brain, spleen, and kidney.
- Decreased by statins.
- Decreases with age starting at fifty years. People aged seventy years have 50 percent less coenzyme Q10 than they did at the age of thirty years.
- Is fat soluble.
- Recycles vitamin E to keep it active.
- Is found in every cell wall.
- Is better absorbed when taken with fats, oils, or vitamin E.
- Helps relieve chronic muscle pain, especially that caused by statins.
- Is beneficial for people with cardiac myopathy.
- Decreases the frequency of arrhythmia.
- Reduces the level of adrenaline.

- Boosts immunity.
- Helps relieve the symptoms of chronic fatigue syndrome when taken in a dosage of 300 mg per day.
- Relieves the adverse effects caused by medications prescribed to treat psychological disorders.
- Facilitates weight loss by increasing the thermogenic activity of muscles.
- Is a powerful antioxidant.
- Can lower elevated systolic blood pressure. However, don't take coenzyme Q10 if you have orthostatic hypotension, which causes you to feel dizzy when you stand up.
- Can block the adverse effects of beta-blockers (feeling tired when you start the b-blockers or when the dose is increased).
- Can decrease the frequency of episodes of angina pectoris.
- Decreases the level of blood sugar in diabetics.
- Decreases the levels of bad cholesterol.
- Decreases the effects of warfarin. It has a physical structure similar to vitamin K, which also reduces the effect of warfarin (Coumadin).
- Protects against cancer.

Coenzyme Q10 is used extensively in Japan; it is the most commonly used drug there. In France, the ginkgo biloba is used the most; but in the USA, it is the codeine.

People with the following conditions or disorders tend to have a low level of coenzyme Q10:

- Diabetes
- Obesity
- Gum disease

- Long-term use of some medications, such as those prescribed to treat psychological disorders.
- Muscular dystrophy (a dosage of 100 mg of coenzyme q10 daily is beneficial).
- Old age
- Heart failure

Sources of Coenzyme Q10 are sardines (the highest level), salmon, liver, meat, and whole grains.

If you are over forty years with any negative factor, take CoQ10 50 mg per day, and if you forgot any supplement I mentioned before, do not forget this one.

L-Carnitine: Cholesterol Reduction Factor

Carnitine, a compound of the amino acids lysine and methionine, transports fatty acids to the mitochondria. Carnitine is produced in the body, and vitamin C is necessary for its synthesis. Children and adolescents may need more carnitine than the body can produce.

Carnitine is found in beef (3 oz contains 90 mg the highest); milk (8 oz contains 4 mg); beans; cereals; honey; vegetables as asparagus, broccoli, and garlic; and legumes.

Like coenzyme Q10, carnitine is found in all cells. Its concentration is particularly high in the brain, heart, and muscles. L-carnitine can cross the brain barrier, giving the mental energy. Carnitine can cross all other cells except the brain. To be activated, carnitine requires vitamin B6. With coenzyme Q10, carnitine drives fatty acids into cells; this decreases the levels of triglyceride and bad cholesterol in the bloodstream and increases the level of good cholesterol.

Bilberry Pills: Improves Retinal Blood and Oxygen Flow

Bilberries are often referred to as the *night vision factor*. They contain flavonoids, anthocyanin, hydroquinone, tannic acid, lutein, and alpha-lipoic acid, which benefits those with Alzheimer's disease.

Remember that bilberries

- improve retinal blood flow;
- protect the collagen in capillaries and decrease the incidence of capillary leaks;
- protect against retinopathy via the action of anthocyanin;
- come in 500 mg, once or twice a day, reduce dose with other blood thinners, act as a urinary tract antiseptic,
- and decrease the incidence of adult macular degeneration.

Alpha-lipoic Acid: Peripheral Neuropathy Factor

This potent antioxidant is found in dark green leafy vegetables, meat, and liver and is consumed as a supplement. The suggested dose of alpha-lipoic acid is 20 to 100 mg per day, although larger doses (for example, 300 mg) are recommended to treat specific health problems such as diabetes.

Alpha-lipoic acid

- recycles vitamins C and E and coenzyme Q10 and restores their antioxidant function,
- relieves peripheral neuritis caused by diabetes,
- benefits those with Parkinson's disease or Alzheimer's disease,
- exerts an antiaging effect by preserving vitamins C and E,
- enhances the action of insulin in people with diabetes, and
- relieves the symptoms of chronic fatigue syndrome.

Ginkgo Biloba: The only OTC macular edema factor (blurry vision), taken by mouth s

The ginkgo biloba is a green leafy tree that can live for more than a thousand years and may attain a height of one hundred feet. The dried leaves of the ginkgo are taken in tablet or capsule form or as a tincture. Ginkgo is a popular diet supplement in Europe. Ginkgos are grown in Japan, China, and Korea. Their leaves contain two important chemical substances: flavonoids, which are potent antioxidants, and terpenoids, which relax the small blood vessels and restore their tone and increase the effects of several blood-thinning agents. In people older than sixty years, the most important effects of ginkgo are those of increasing memory and the ability to learn, preventing nerve injury from oxidative damage (a factor in those with Alzheimer's disease or another type of brain degeneration), exerting an anti-inflammatory effect, and lowering high blood pressure. Ginkgo also improves circulation in the legs and relieves the leg pain and cramping of the calf muscles that can occur after walking. If you have problems with the circulation in your legs, be sure to see your doctor, especially if you have diabetes because early treatment can prevent infection and the need for amputation. The improvement in circulation caused by ginkgo also benefits the eyes, especially the retinas. It helps relieve macular edema—the only OTC drug that can reduce macular edema by mouth. Add to that, there is no known prescription medicine that can do its action yet without bad complication. Take one pill of 80 mg at night (a fact to which I can attest from personal experience) and you will see the results in the morning,. Use it for few days till you improve, then stop, repeat if the blurry vision comes back. The benefits of ginkgo are usually noticed within a few weeks, except in those with macular edema. In my case, macular edema improved within twenty-four hours after I had taken the first dose of ginkgo, and I also noticed a reduction in glare. I took ginkgo with a supplement containing vitamin B complex that included vitamin B6 and vitamin C. Eighty milligrams of ginkgo can be given three times daily to people with severe dementia.

Cautions about Ginkgo

Although ginkgo confers many benefits, be aware of the following cautions about this powerful supplement:

- It has not been shown to benefit children.
- It is an anticoagulant (a blood thinner), so if you take a medication that thins your blood, please check with your doctor before you take ginkgo or internal bleeding (for example, in the stomach) can result.

- It should not be taken for at least three days before you undergo surgery, especially the eye and the brain, or excessive bleeding can develop.
- It can increase the action of anticonvulsant medications.
- It can increase the action of oral contraceptives.
- It may be helpful in relieving scotoma (poor central vision), research has suggested.

Zinc

Zinc is often referred to as the *eye health factor*. Every cell in your body needs it.

Here are some facts about this essential element:

- Oysters and beef are high in zinc.
- Zinc is essential for the formation of chlorophyll and carbohydrates in plants.
- It is needed to ensure the functioning of three hundred enzymes in the body.
- Unlike calcium or magnesium, zinc cannot be stored in the body.
- Your body needs 15 mg of zinc daily (or 30 mg daily if you have diabetic eye disease).
- More than 1,000 mg per day of zinc is toxic.
- Zinc promotes wound healing when applied as a skin ointment.
- It improves immune system functioning.
- It benefits vision.
- It decreases vascular retinopathy.

- It decreases capillary degeneration; you may avoid the high complication retinal laser surgery.
- A high intake of zinc can reduce your levels of copper and manganese, so if you take supplementary zinc, be sure to consume a sufficient amount of copper and manganese in food or take a daily supplement (such as Centrum) that contains those elements.

Zinc is found in meat, fish, spinach, and eggs.

Magnesium: Diabetes Prevention Factor

Part of hundreds of cellular enzymes, this is almost needed for most body functions; it is one of the most important metals in the body. Fifty percent of magnesium is in the bones and teeth.

The daily value for magnesium is 75 to 100 mg.

Remember these facts about magnesium:

- It is required for energy production and sugar control.
- It is a natural calcium channel blocker to reduce blood pressure.
- It is necessary for bone formation, muscle function, and digestion.
- It prevents tissue calcification.
- It may help dissolve kidney stones when taken with vitamin B6.
- It protects against and inhibits the progression of osteoporosis.
- It decreases the levels of bad cholesterol.
- It is important in calcium, potassium, phosphorus, and vitamin C metabolism.
- It helps you sleep.

A deficiency of magnesium (which can be caused by diarrhea, vomiting, alcohol consumption, or a high-protein, high-calcium, high-carbohydrate diet) produces insomnia, irritability, diabetes, asthma, hypertension, and cardiac arrhythmia.

Magnesium is found in halibut, almonds, and soybeans.

It occurs in high concentrations in meat, fruits, vegetables, brown rice, chamomile, licorice, and peppermint.

Seventy percent of US citizens' diet does not meet the percent DV of magnesium. Remember, calcium alone can't treat osteoporosis, but calcium and magnesium can, in a ratio of three to one (for example: 1,200 mg calcium, and 400 mg magnesium per day)

Calcium: The Bone Factor

Calcium is often called the *bone factor*, but it is found in all cell membranes and hormones. It is a structural part of the skeletal system and teeth and is important for

- each heartbeat,
- nerve conduction,
- the functioning of the central nervous system (that is, the brain and spinal cord),
- muscle contraction and function,
- blood clotting,
- maintaining blood pressure and blood vessel tone,
- cell metabolism in soft tissues,
- protection against polyps in the colon,

- reducing the levels of bad cholesterol, and
- producing energy.

Ingested iron and sugar and a high-fat, high-protein diet reduce calcium absorption. Calcium is deposited on the surface of bones and can be recalled from that storage when needed. However, certain conditions can deplete calcium reserves. A calcium deficiency can be caused by the following:

- Poor intake of calcium-containing foods, milk, cheese, and calcium-fortified soy milk.
- Poor calcium absorption, which can occur after an intestinal operation or as a result of aging or low vitamin D, antireflux medications (protein pump inhibitors), pancreatitis, and metastases of tumors.
- Alcoholism, because alcohol has a diuretic effect and calcium is lost via excessive urination. Symptoms of low calcium (hypocalcemia) start if the total calcium in the blood is less than 8.2 mg/dl. (Normal blood calcium is 8.7 to 10.4 mg/dl.)
- If the blood level of calcium is less than 8.2 mg/dl, it is low; but since half the calcium is attached to the blood protein albumin, the body really works with 4.5 mg/dl called the ionized calcium. Symptoms start if the ionized calcium is less than 4 mg/dl: tingling of feet, fingers, lips, and tongue; spasm of feet, hands, and cheek muscles; hyperactive reflexes (Chvostek sign)—if you tap over the facial nerve located in front of the ear, midpart, twitching of the perioral muscles (lips) occur; cardiac arrhythmia and electrocardiogram changes.
- the treatment, after proper and fast evaluation; is by intravenous calcium.

- note that Any patient undergoing parathyroid resection may develop hypocalcaemia, and seizures and cardiac disasters may follow.

Hypercalcemia

It happens in most cases. If the parathyroid hormone is secreted in excess by a parathyroid gland tumor, removal of the tumor or parathyroid gland usually is curative.

It also can be a sign of vitamin D toxicity.

Symptoms:

- Usually less than hypocalcemia, high calcium gives symptoms if it is over 14 mg/dl.
- Nausea, vomiting, stomach pain, drowsiness, depression, and polyuria
- It can give high blood pressure and low pulse.
- At higher levels it can give coma and death.

Calcium Supplement Dose

The recommended dosage of calcium is 1,200 to 1,500 per day, and consuming 1,000 mg daily is recommended for those older than seventy years. Calcium is found in most foods. Seventy-five percent of calcium is consumed in dairy products such as milk, cheese, and yogurt; fruits, vegetables, meat, fish, and beans are the food sources for the remaining 25 percent. The amount of calcium that you need daily is determined by your age, the rate at which your body absorbs calcium from various sources, the amount of calcium consumed, and the types of calcium-containing food ingested

Consider adding the calcium-rich foods listed below, with their respective calcium values, to your diet.

1 cup of tofu: 250 mg
3 oz of canned fish: 200 mg
3 oz of canned sardines: 200 mg
1 oz of cheddar cheese: 200 mg
1 oz of cottage cheese: 155 mg
1 oz of Swiss cheese: 272 mg
1 cup of whole milk: 300 mg
1 cup of skim milk: 300 mg
3 oz of yogurt: 300 mg
1 cup of fortified soy milk: 250 mg
5 dried figs, 200 mg (figs has tryptophan, potassium, fiber)

Foods with calcium, but not for disease treatment:

½ cup of beans: 60 mg one cup of broccoli: 40 mg
1 orange (medium size): 30 mg

Calcium can also be ingested in tablets that contain calcium citrate, calcium carbonate, or calcium glaciate. Of those forms, calcium citrate is absorbed most efficiently because it is acidic. Calcium carbonate can be taken on an empty stomach so that gastric acid improves its absorption. Calcium gluconate is absorbed least effectively. Coral calcium is a good source of calcium, but it is often contaminated with toxic substances such as lead or mercury. People

THE MEDITERRANEAN FARMER'S SON'S DIET

with lactose intolerance, which is common in Asians, blacks, and people of Mediterranean descent, can consume their calcium in fortified juices, soy milk enriched with calcium, lactose-free milk, vegetables, legumes, or fortified cereals.

Boron

The daily value of this trace element, which is found in fruits and vegetables, is 3 mg in healthy individuals and up to 15 mg in those with a disease such as osteoporosis.

Boron helps the body conserve calcium and magnesium, decreases the risk for osteoporosis, and benefits memory.

Potassium

We need 3,500 mg of potassium per day.

Here are some facts to remember about potassium, the recommended daily value of which is 4,000 mg:

- It is important in maintaining electrolyte balance.
- It is essential for muscle contraction and nerve conduction.
- It is lost via vomiting, diarrhea, and increased urination.

A potassium deficiency can cause

- electrocardiographic abnormalities;
- paralytic ileus (belly distended without mechanical blockage, just temporarily paralyzed intestine);

- alkalosis;
- arrhythmia; and
- cardiac arrest (in people with a severe potassium deficiency).

The following foods are high in potassium:

Oranges
Bananas (the highest, up to 500 mg in a large banana)
Lemons
Avocados
Nuts
Beans
Dates
Raisins
All leafy green vegetables

High potassium diet if not contraindicated like in renal failure cases reduces strokes and as good as a baby aspirin.

Something Called the Poly Pill: It Is Very Interesting

The Polly Pill

UK researchers examined more than four hundred thousand participants. They estimated that such pill will reduce heart disease and stroke risks on people over fifty-five by 80 percent, and they are concentrating on people who already have risks like heart disease, high blood pressure, and diabetes.

The magic pill contains baby aspirin, statins, diuretics, beta-blocker, ACE inhibitors, and folic acid for 1 mg.

The review of the study shows that statins prevented 61 percent heart disease and 16 percent of stroke.

Blood-pressure-lowering medication, which is the ACE inhibitors, prevents 46 percent of heart attacks and 63 percent of strokes.

Folic acid, which is an anti homocysteine, prevents 15 percent of heart attacks and 25 percent of stroke.

Aspirin prevented 32 percent of heart attacks and 16 percent of strokes.

They calculated that all in all, it will reduce 80 percent of the heart attack as well as strokes. The poly pill is advised for people over fifty-five years or older to avoid heart attacks and strokes, especially those who have signs of heart disease, but more study is needed.

Some of the people who take aspirin really cannot tolerate it. They may bleed from the stomach as well as the brain; they may develop ulcer, so you might to be careful with this and just take baby aspirin for 81 mg.

Now some people have no high blood pressure; that's why the minimal amount of ACE inhibitor will be used.

The folic acid relates its effect to neutralizing the homocysteine effect. The homocysteine is known to damage the inside, which is called the endothelium tissues in the vessels.

The statins reduce cholesterol as well as it reduces inflammation of the vessels.

In my opinion the six medications are good; the question is, do you need them all or not? It depends on your situation. People who have very low blood pressure do not have to take blood pressure medication. But don't forget that these medication sometimes given to people who have protein urea.

When it comes to aspirin, it definitely has an anti-inflammatory action and is well-known and agreed by all doctors that we need it. Some people are allergic to it or cannot tolerate it. I suggest you take vitamin E for 400 mg to 600 mg a day; this is an antioxidant and can give a little blood thinning. Vitamin C and omega-3 can do the same.

If you have other diseases, you may need Plavix if you have previous clotting problems.

You can exchange some of these medications with less effective but also less injurious of supplements or foods. Suppose you have liver disease and you want to take a statin medications like Lipitor and Crestor, these medications can cause liver toxicity. In this case you have to go for vitamin E, omega-3, niacin, garlic pills, and increase some foods like carrots, apples, onions, fresh garlic, and high-fiber diets.

When you take beta-blockers, it is suggested with ace inhibitors, it is a high blood pressure medications too.

ACE inhibitors, these are the good ones; in very small doses they can reduce proteinurea from the kidney, improve heart and retina function with minimal postural hypotension, especially if taken before sleep in a small dose, for example, 2.5 mg Altace, or 2. 5 mg of Accupril. When it comes to diuretics, especially if you do not have any other diseases and you have a systolic type of hypertension, this will be perfect to reduce mild systolic pressure if it's in 140-145.

The African Americans, as well as the Asians respond very well to diuretics because a lot of them have systolic type of hypertension.

When it comes to aspirin, again you can change it with vitamin E if you cannot tolerate it or even go with medically prescribed medications.

I want to talk more about the poly pill: it has six components, and it is the one that can give you eleven years more in your life without a stroke or heart attack.

1. Aspirin

Baby aspirin for 81 mg—you can find it as in Ecotrin, which is an aspirin plus antacid. Or as St. Joseph aspirin, which is sublingual. I prefer a noncoated aspirin since the coat may contain aluminum, which causes Alzheimer's. Also, it bypasses the stomach. By the way, aspirin can give acidity and reflux and even bleeding in the stomach, but it's less if taken sublingually. Baby aspirin is an over-the-counter drug. By the way, if you smoke one cigarette, it can destroy the effectiveness of aspirin for twenty-four hours.

2. Folic Acid

Folic acid is good for the heart and the blood; it works against homocysteine, which is a separate factor as bad as cholesterol. Folic acid of 1 mg a day can neutralize it.

3. Statins

If your cholesterol is not high, it is suggested to take a small dose of a statin because of its anti-inflammatory effect, and as I am going to say in another book, this function of the statins may be even more important than reducing the cholesterol itself. CRP is a test to check for the inflammation factor in the blood. Statins reduce inflammation that means it can reduce the clogging of your vessels. It also can reduce triglycerides in diabetics.

4. ACE Inhibitors

These are high blood pressure medications, which has other additional benefits. It helps the retinopathy leaks. It helps the heart, and it improves its circulation. It helps the leaking kidney because it cuts down on the protein urea when the protein passes through the kidney excessively, which is supposed to be zero; protein in the urine can give the kidney problems later on.

5. Beta-blockers

The beta-blockers are given to most heart attack patients with high pulse conditions; by the way, protein urea and beta-blockers are checked during a life insurance examination because if you are taking it, this means you have previous heart problem.

6. Diuretics or Water Pills

It is given for multi conditions.

Please notice that beta-blockers, statins, diuretics, and ACE inhibitors are given under a doctor's supervision. The poly pill doctors want to give people over fifty or younger with negative factors.

When it comes to aspirin, if you can tolerate aspirin, you should take it after meals. If you have a history of heart problem or transient ischemic attacks, where you lose your vision temporarily or lose your balance, you should see the doctor. Now your body is warning you, have help now. Your doctor will increase the aspirin dose or add to aspirin something like Plavix after doing some workup to rule out other things. The best doctor to go to in this case is a cardiologist or a neurologist or a vascular surgeon.

Aspirin may be indicated now. In fact, I like to carry one 81 mg in my pocket in case I get a problem in the car or at work. An aspirin can reduce heart pains and strokes, and if it happens, it will give you time to reach the emergency room alive. Try to go to a hospital, a trauma center, or a large hospital unless you are too far from that type of hospital.

Water

Molecules of water are composed of one oxygen atom and two hydrogen atoms. Water (H_2O) has several different forms, which include clouds, water, ice, and steam. Water is essential for all forms of life. Pure water is colorless in small amounts and blue in large quantities. Even with all the advances of the modern world, one billion people are still drinking dirty water. Pure water has a faint color.

All life requires water, and nothing lives long without it. Here are some facts to remember about water, which we need in abundance every day:

- Some types of water have a taste; for example, ocean water is salty, and spring water is fresh and clean but may contain extra calcium. Hard water has high levels of calcium and magnesium, and chemically softened water (from which as much calcium and magnesium as possible have been removed) is usually obtained by adding potassium or sodium.

- Even today, with all the technologic benefits that many of us enjoy, one billion people still drink dirty water. Running water may be infected with the bacterium *Escherichia coli*, which lives in the colon and is transmitted by contamination with human waste.
- Ocean water is salty.
- Pure spring water is fresh and clean but may contain extra calcium.
- Hard water is high in calcium and magnesium, which can be counteracted by the addition of a water softener such as potassium or sodium.
- When you have hard water, soap does not lather easily and leaves a film on whatever it touches, so using soft water may be preferable.
- Running water may contain *Escherichia coli,* a bacterium that thrives in human waste and can contaminate a water supply.
- Both mineral water, which may contain sodium, and distilled water are okay to drink.

For good health, try to drink eight ounce of water eight times per day (drink more water during or after exercise or if you are perspiring). Remember that when you perspire, you lose sodium and your risk for hyponatremia (a low level of sodium in the bloodstream) can increase. However, hyponatremia can also occur if you drink too much water because you then lose electrolytes including sodium via excessive urination.

City drinking water contains fluoride (usually 1 to 3 mg/l), which is good for the teeth especially of children. If the level of fluoride in drinking water exceeds 4 mg/l, then it becomes a health hazard and may cause tooth enamel damage, bone cancer, fractures, skeletal fluorosis, calcifications in the knees with pain.

During exercise, you must increase the amount of water and salt that you drink. In 2002, a young female athlete who was running a marathon collapsed and died because she lost too much sodium by perspiring excessively, and low blood pressure developed. If your sodium level reaches 118 mg/l (normal is 135 to 145 mg/l), low blood pressure and collapse may ensue. To treat high blood pressure, you should eat a low-sodium diet, but to prevent very low blood pressure, like the level that occurred in that marathon runner, you need the sodium in diet. For that reason, many beverages designed for athletes are fortified to prevent the loss of essential elements.

If you drink one cup of coffee, then you should drink one to two cups of water to reduce the degree of dehydration that coffee causes.

Drink a cup of water before breakfast. If you suffer from constipation, then drink two cups of water and eat a high-fiber food. The excess water will work as a stool softener.

If you drink a cup of tea or beer, then drink a cup of water to combat the dehydrating effects of excessive urination.

The various types of drinking water include distilled water and mineral water, which contains sodium. I suggest drinking one eight-ounce cup of water eight to ten times daily and more if you are exercising. Sweating during exercise removes sodium from the body, and a condition called *hyponatremia*—low sodium in the bloodstream can develop. However, drinking too much water causes excessive urination, which results in the depletion of sodium, potassium, calcium, and other elements from the bloodstream. Sodium is the mineral that is lost first when excessive urination occurs, and symptoms of hyponatremia can develop. If your normal sodium level is above 145 and quickly decreases to 132, you may experience dizziness that increases if excessive urination continues.

Drinking Water

Drinking water is truly the fountain of health. Let's review the types of water that are available to us and consider their differences.

Bottled Water

Bottled water (distilled water, sparkling water, fortified water) lacks fluoride, which is naturally present in groundwater and is necessary for healthy, cavity-free teeth. Bottled water is usually deficient in calcium and magnesium. Processed municipal water may be fluorinated and may contain small doses of supplements such as potassium and calcium. Here are a few examples of commercially available bottled water.

Dasani

Dasani is local water from municipal water that has been filtered via reverse osmosis and supplemented with traces of minerals (potassium and calcium).

Seltzer

Seltzer (pH 7.5) is alkaline. It is high in minerals. For example, each liter of seltzer contains 17 mg of calcium and 13 mg of magnesium.

Flavored Noncarbonated Water (Various Brands)

Noncarbonated bottled water, which is available in a variety of flavors with or without natural or artificial sweeteners, may contain supplements such as vitamin E, vitamin B1, potassium, calcium, and/or sodium. Most flavored bottled water brands are low in carbohydrates and calories or are calorie free.

Aquafina

Aquafina is noncarbonated tap water that has been extensively purified, and most minerals are usually removed during the process.

Evian

Evian is a brand of spring water from the French Alps. It is slightly acidic and contains calcium, carbohydrates, magnesium, and potassium. Like all purified water, Evian is without pollutants such as lead and radon.

Municipal (City) Water

Some municipal types of water are good, some are bad, and some are in-between. Check with your city to determine whether your municipal water supply provides you with pure, clean drinking water.

Who should not take too much or restrict water?

- People with congestive heart failure.
- Those who have fluid in their lungs.

- People with ascites—that is, fluid in the belly around the stomach.
- Those with kidney disease. The kidneys filter toxins and waste products and discharge them in urine. In people with kidney failure, drinking excess water can overload the circulatory system and cause acute lung edema and heart problems.

Spices

Flavorful spices have enhanced foods and beverages for thousands of years, and in many cultures, their medicinal value has been recognized as well. Let's revisit some herbs and spices long known to improve health and prevent *disease*.

Black Seed: The Immunity Factor

Black seed (*Nigel sativa*, black cumin seed, blessed seeds, seeds of blessing, *habit al-baraka* [Arabic]) has been used as a spice for more than two thousand years. Found in the tomb of Tutankhamen, black seed was thought to help him in his second life. This spice, which is found in the Middle East, Turkey, and India is harvested from a blue-flowered plant. Black seed, which is mentioned in the Bible, was referred to by the Prophet Mohammed as "blessed seeds" that could heal all diseases except death.

Black seed has 100 nutritional components, contains beneficial oils (35 percent), contains essential fatty acids (50 percent), and contains volatile oils (5 percent) that act as an antihistamine and dilate the bronchi.

Each 5-mm black seed contains about one hundred nutrients, such as calcium, potassium, zinc, magnesium, vitamin A, vitamin B1, vitamin B2, niacin, and vitamin C.

Here are a few additional facts about black seed:

- One teaspoon weighs 3 grams and contains 12 calories (six of which are from oil).
- It contains eight of the nine essential amino acids.
- It contains unsaturated (good) fatty acids, including omega-3 and omega-6.
- It is consumed as whole seeds, ground seeds, a paste or oil.
- It improves the immune system functioning, especially in people with an autoimmune disease.
- It helps heal eczema and psoriasis.
- It relieves the symptoms of asthma and bronchitis.
- In Jordan, research has shown that black seed exerts an antileukemic, anti-inflammatory, and anticancer effects and is especially prophylactic against prostate cancer.
- It is an anthelmintic.
- It exerts an antibiotic effect.
- It can stimulate the menstrual cycle.
- It increases the milk flow in lactating women.
- Its powder or oil can be added to bread, onions, coffee, or tea.
- One teaspoon of black seed oil or one 50 to 75 mg capsule of black seed taken with meals for a few months increases the luster of hair and nails.
- Black seed can be added to honey or ginger.
- It reduces the levels of bad cholesterol.

- It contains sterols (including B-sterol, which is anticarcinogenic).
- Research indicates that it impedes malignant tumor growth and metastasis.
- It improves digestion.
- It stimulates bone morrow and the immune system to increase the levels of interferons needed to repel viral and bacterial infections.
- It can increase the activity of helper T cells to suppressor T cells by 72 percent if given 1 g twice a day for four weeks. The research was done by Dr. Eked in Saudi Arabia showed that black seed increases immunity.
- It stimulates the release of prostaglandin E1.
- It decreases the body's overreaction to autoimmune disease. It decreases inflammation and increases immunity to allergic antigens. It works like interferon but without the complications associated with interferon use. Interferon increases the host resistance to viruses and tumor by improving immunity.
- It relieves insomnia and induces relaxation.
- Mix one tablespoon of black seed oil or paste and one teaspoon of honey, then eat with whole grain bread.
- Black seed is beneficial for people with diabetes because it contains antioxidants and good fats and because it stimulates the immune system to ward off infections.
- It is a component of the Mediterranean diet and is added to fried or grilled foods, rice, cheese, fish, meat, and bread stuffing.
- The taste of black seed can be masked by royal jelly or honey.

Curcumin: The Alzheimer's Factor

Hippocrates said, "Let food be thy medicine and medicine be thy food." Curcumin (*karkum* in Arabic) is extracted from turmeric roots. It is a major ingredient in curry to which it imparts a yellow color. Curcumin has been recognized for hundreds of years as a treatment for toothache and a digestive aid.

India has the lowest incidence of Alzheimer's disease in the world, which is due to curcumin in the curry that is a dietary staple there. Recently, other researchers have reached that same conclusion.

Remember these facts about curcumin:

- It exerts an anti-inflammatory effect that relieves the symptoms of arthritis and some pulmonary diseases.
- It is beneficial for people with a neurologic disease (primarily Alzheimer's disease).
- It protects against the development of autoimmune diseases, cardiovascular diseases, liver diseases, and diabetes.
- It reduces the levels of bad cholesterol and increases the level of good cholesterol without causing the adverse effects produced by drugs such as rosuvastatin (Crestor).
- It is a detoxifying agent; for example, it prevents the absorption of pesticides in the intestine.
- My recommended dosage is one 500 mg capsule of curcumin three times daily.
- It protects against cancers of the colon, skin, and breast by inhibiting the growth and metastasis of malignant cells.

- It works primarily in the liver, where (like the drug ezetimibe [Zetia]) it prevents the absorption of cholesterol and bile acids in the small bowel.
- It increases the action of CD4 and T helper lymphocytes, both of which improve immunity.
- It can be added to ice cream, bread, cakes, cheese, and tea and used as a food color.
- It exerts an antiamyloid effect, which may be the most important action of this spice. Curcumin reduces the buildup of plaque (beta-amyloid) in the brain and prevents the formation of new plaque (this type of plaques are part of or the cause of Alzheimer's disease). Remember that curry and curcumin are used extensively in India, which has the lowest incidence of Alzheimer's disease in the world.

Don't ingest curcumin if you have jaundice caused by blockage of the common bile duct or if you take the blood thinner warfarin (Coumadin).

Curry powder, which is used in drinks, tea, and yogurt and is added to beans, meat, and rice contains

- turmeric root (which supplies the color and is the primary ingredient in most curries);
- cumin, which protects against infection;
- fenugreek, which is good for people with diabetes;
- mustard;
- chili powder;
- salt; nutmeg; and
- ginger.

Cumin: The Flatulence Factor

Cumin is used extensively as a seasoning in India, Africa, and the Middle East. The flowers and seeds (yellow or white) of the plant *Cumin cyminum* are used to make this fragrant spice. Cumin, which has a strong aroma, is added to bread in France, to cheese in Holland, to curry in India, and with chili powder, to meat in the American Southwest. It is a good source of iron and potassium, and it contains some fiber. One tablespoon of cumin contains 3 mg of iron (20 percent of the daily value), 100 mg of potassium, and 1 g of fiber.

It is added to cauliflower to reduce flatulence.

Rose Hips

Rose hips contain flavonoids as well as vitamins C and E.
They help relieve the symptoms of cold and flu.
They induce a feeling of relaxation. Add it to chamomile and anise.

CHAPTER 8

Staying Healthy the Easy Way
(Surda, My Village Doses)

A healthful lifestyle is more than a good diet and regular medical checkups. It's a long-term plan that provides you with the best safeguards for achieving and maintaining good health. In this chapter, we'll revisit foods and nutrients that are essential to good health, and we'll consider some lifestyle tips that are part of a healthful way of living, day by day and over time.

Live a Healthful Lifestyle

Catch a Few Sun Rays

Sunshine is essential to the body's natural production of vitamin D, and evidence suggests that brief exposure to the sun when you are not wearing sunscreen can help to alleviate depression. Exposure to sunshine for forty-five minutes even in the winter increases the level of serotonin and decreases the craving for any food.

Keep Lean

Avoiding overweight is more than a sign of self-control; it is essential to good health. Maintaining a healthful weight will help you reach your nineties.

Increase Your Level of Good Cholesterol

To increase your level of good cholesterol without prescription medication:

- The farmer's diet way, eat four to six halves walnut daily (it works like niacin to raise the good cholesterol), with no side effects like flushing).
- Also, to increase good cholesterol, some people eat three fresh garlic pods before sleep daily (cut them in halves and swallow them with water like pills).
- Take onion, apple pectin, carrots, and olive oil.
- The cheapest way is to exercise.
- The most expensive way is to take a few weeks' vacation.
- The farmer's son's life extender, the extra virgin olive oil, take two to three table spoonfull a day (take it with bread, cheese or any food which fits your weight, to avoid its acidic taste in the throat) at the same time reduce the meat and margarine fats. although olive oil has a definite lowering effect on bad cholesterol, and increase the good cholesterol, I BELIEVE it has other functions which Iam trying to prove

Other Good Habits

Exercise—it is the best and cheapest way to stay healthy.

Take a supplement containing both omega-3 fatty acids and vitamin C.

Follow a high-fiber diet that is low in saturated fat.

Avoid dietary *trans* fats.

Take a vitamin B complex supplement to ensure that your diet contains enough nicotinic acid and niacin. Niacin is high in beef liver, chicken breast, and tuna (14 mg per 3.5 oz) and to a less extent in whole grains, peanut, and carrot. Take apple pectin, garlic, and oregano; they reduce bad cholesterol and improve the good to bad cholesterol ratio.

Eat These Foods as Often as Possible

Each day, eat a reasonable amount of as many of the foods listed below as you can. Divide your daily food intake into three 500-calorie meals plus two 250-calorie snacks.

- Olive oil one to two teaspoonfuls (thirty calories per teaspoon) with whole grains or added to salad one or more a day; olive oil is a life extender.
- Oranges and limes, which are high in vitamin C and potassium.
- Pear and eggplants, which are high in fiber and low in calorie.
- Carrots, which are high in vitamins A and B and in the antioxidant beta-carotene (which assists in tissue repair).
- Macadamia nuts, which are high in monounsaturated fatty acids like olive oil.

- Pistachio nuts. They contain high polyunsaturated fat—the good fat.
- Corn and squash, which contain fiber and vitamin A.
- Okra, which is high in fiber and magnesium.
- Asparagus, which helps to prevent the formation of kidney stones, contains rutin, which strengthens capillaries and reduce one small vein leak of fluid. This is good for diabetic retinopathy and leg edema.
- Figs, which are high in calcium and fiber, for those who are allergic to milk.
- Papayas, which contain more beta-carotene than does any other fruit.
- Almonds, which are high in vitamin E and magnesium. Good for diabetes.
- Raisins, which are high in iron and good for blood formation. And resveratrol, which is good for the heart
- Apricots, which are a good source of vitamin A for tissue repair and effective immune system function.

Add Essential Vitamins, Minerals, and Nutrients to Your Diet

The adage "moderation in all things" also applies to vitamin supplements. Here is information about the amounts of vitamins and minerals that are needed every day.

- Vitamin A of no more than 5,000 IU daily unless a different dosage is prescribed by your doctor. Vitamin A accumulates in the body, and too high a dosage can build up to a toxic level over time. It is for eye health. It is the orange color of the carrots and is high in prunes, sweet potato, fresh thyme, and cantaloupe.

- Beta-carotene of 15,000 IU per day, which is found in the same sources as vitamin A, exerts an antioxidant effect and promotes tissue repair. They are essential for eye health and can give vitamin A.

- The following B vitamins, when needed, improve circulation, hormone production, blood formation, cell division and function, and enzyme production:

  B1: 100 to 300 mg per day for nerves' health and the tremors associated with alcohol withdrawal

  B2: riboflavin, 50 to 200 mg for migraine headache and antiviral and antibacterial effect

  Niacin: 100 mg for people with diabetes but up to 2,000 mg per day for nondiabetic individuals. It reduces high triglycerides and increases good cholesterol.

  Nicotinamide: 100 mg. It functions like niacin, it can give flushing and postural hypotension.

  B6: 50 mg is good for first trimester nausea and vomiting. It is good for nerve health and diabetes control.

  B12: 50 to 300 IU. It is the nerve cell health and the antihallucination in the elderly factor. It is good for brain nerve cells, the nerves, and red blood cell function.

Biotin: 300 mcg. The retina energy factor, biotin, (when taken in large doses) can prevent diabetic neuropathy. Biotin should be taken in a dose of 30, 50, 100, or 200 mcg per day to treat diabetic neuropathy or 2.5 mg per day to treat brittle nails.

- Folic acid: 400 mcg to 1 mg. It blocks homocysteine, a separate inflammatory factor, and helps reduce cardiovascular disease.
- Vitamin C alleviates bruising, strengthens capillary cell walls, and improves tissue oxygenation. It is a good free radical scavenger, increases circulation, improves immune system function, and decreases the level of histamine. Take 500 to 1,000 mg twice daily.
- Vitamin D 400 IU—the bone health factor.
- Vitamin E 400 IU. (If this vitamin is taken instead of aspirin to prevent stomach irritation and gastric ulcers, add 800 mcg of vitamin E to your diet). Vitamin E of 400 mcg twice a day promotes healthy skin, immune system function, circulation, and blood thinning. A deficiency in vitamin E may increase the risk for breast cancer.
- Potassium 4,000 mg keeps body pH in-line; it is important for muscle and nerve function. It is high in apricots, banana, lime, avocado, beans and nuts, and cabbage. Do not use if you have a renal failure.
- Calcium 1,500 mg. It is the bone builder and is good for heart and muscle function.
- Chromium 150 mcg, which increases insulin sensitivity and decreases the use of muscle as a protein source for energy in people with insulin resistance. 10 to 150 mcg?

- It stabilizes sugar level in the blood. It is high in beef liver, onion, and romaine lettuce, but the best source is a polyvitamin Centrum pill. It has 150 mcg, which is a good dose.
- Copper 2 mg is good for bone and collagen tissue health.
- Iron 250 mg is good for anemia caused by excessive bleeding like heavy menstruation.
- Manganese 10 to 30 mg. It is for the health of nerves, bones, thyroid, and is an enzyme used by the mitochondria in each cell as anti-free radicals. It is high in pineapples, chickpeas, brown rice, and whole grains.
- Selenium 70 mcg gives part of enzymes as antioxidants; it is highest in Brazil nuts, which is 750 mcg per ounce, beef, and tuna for 50 mcg per ounce.
- Zinc 30 mg is necessary for protein synthesis, collagen formation, tissue repair, and sex hormones and immune system function.
- Magnesium 400 mg is for bone health and blood sugar control. It is a natural calcium channel blocker or lowers high blood pressure. It is high in pumpkin seeds, sesame seeds, soybeans, salmon, and spinach.

Be sure that your diet also contains the following:

- Coenzyme Q10 improves the oxygenation of cells. A dose of 30 to 100 mg is good for myalgia, including the myalgia caused by statins.
- Pectin 100 mg (apple skin) is the cholesterol and constipation factor.

- L-carnitine 80 mg increases the level of good cholesterol and reduces cholesterol by pushing it inside the cells to be used for energy.
- Beta-carotene is found in pink-colored fruits like prunes, tomato, and cantaloupe. It exerts an antioxidant effect and promotes tissue repair.
- Genistein, which is an isoflavone and antioxidant that is found in soybeans. Eat soybeans. Genistein may stop the formation of new blood vessels in malignant tumors.
- Phytochemicals present in citrus fruits and beans, which give plants color, flavor, and a natural resistance to some diseases. In humans, phytochemicals decrease the risk for cancer, lower blood pressure, and exert an anti-free radical effect.
- Alpha-lipoic acid 100 mg helps to alleviate peripheral neuropathy and can reduce the risk for kidney disease in people with diabetes by lowering the level of a sugar by-product called fructosamine. It is good for diabetic retinopathy and polyneuropathy. It is an antioxidant, which can regenerate the vitamins E and C. This is high in liver and kidney meats, broccoli, and potatoes.

Enjoy Healthful Foods, Flavorful Spices, and Tasty Low-Calorie Snacks

These healthful foods, herbs, and nutrients can be a part of your everyday diet added to other dishes or enjoyed as an occasional snack.

- Brazil nuts, which contain hundred times more selenium than does any other nut. Brazil nuts exert an anti-free radical effect, provide protection against prostate cancer and heart disease, and improve circulation. They are a good source of essential amino acids, nicotinamide, and pantothenic acid (the antistress acid). Brazil nuts may retard aging and assist in cell reproduction.

- Garlic, which is a natural antibiotic, enhances immunity, exerts a powerful antioxidant effect, lowers high blood pressure, and reduces the amount of fat in the bloodstream.

- Cabbage, which contains flavonoids that are not destroyed by cooking also has chromium.

- Citrus fruits, the potassium, vitamin C, calcium, and the natural fructose source.

- Broccoli, which blocks the activity of carcinogens and neutralizes their effects in the intestine.

- Green tea, which contains catechins such as epigallocatechin gallate or EGCG. Green tea may inhibit the growth of cancer of the breast, stomach, and pancreas.

- Grape seed extract and grape seed oil, which contain proanthocyanidin, are good for chronic venous insufficiency and spider naevi and exert an antioxidant effect. Grape seeds heal oozing capillaries in the retina and under the skin and improve the strength of collagen, which strengthens blood vessel walls. It also has resveratrol, which dilates the coronaries and stops cancer cells from dividing and block enzymes needed for the cancer cell to grow.

- Thyme, which contains thirty times more antioxidants than does a medium-size red apple. Thyme antagonizes nitrous oxide, which is a harmful free radical.

- Oregano, which contains a level of antioxidants as thyme taken as dried. Zaatar leaves are eaten fresh with olive oil. Oregano and thyme are called the intelligent factors or information storage factors in the brain. Eat it daily. It is low in calorie and very nutritious.
- Black grapes have more resveratrol than the seeds, a substance that increases nitric acid, which dilates the blood vessels of and nourishes the heart. Remember that *nitric acid* is good, but *nitrous acid* is bad for your health.
- Pomegranates, which are very high in antioxidants (in fact, higher than green tea in antioxidant content). Pomegranates protect against cancer, Alzheimer's disease, and atherosclerosis.
- Kiwifruit, which contains a high level of vitamin E and lutein—a substance that improves night vision.
- Parsley, high in chlorophyll, vitamin C, and antioxidants, which neutralize carcinogens in the bloodstream as does broccoli in the intestine.
- Bilberries, which contains anthocyanin, prevent night blindness and protect against retinopathy.

These substances are also essential to good health:

- L-carnitine, which decreases the total cholesterol level and increases the level of good cholesterol by driving molecules of fat into cells and thus removing fat from the bloodstream.
- Ginkgo biloba, which contains terpenoids that restore the tone of and relax the small arterial vessels in the legs and retina. It also contains flavonoids that are antioxidants. Ginkgo

can improve macular edema more effectively than can any over-the-counter medication. There are no prescription drugs available for macular edema except cortisone injections, and it has high complications.

Avoid Foods That May Harm Your Health

The following foods may adversely affect your health:

- Aspartame, which is made of aspartic acids, phenylalanine, and methanol syrup. It is probably the methanol by-products of aspartame that cause problems with vision and memory. Replace with one teaspoonful of honey, it is fifteen calories.
- All processed sugars, such as table sugar, brown sugar, or high-fructose corn syrup and raw cane sugar. Instead, replace them with fruits, juices, complex carbohydrates from beans and nuts, and honey for coffee or teas.
- Cola and Sprite. Instead, take water or juice.
- Beef. Instead, choose goat meat or chicken (white meat).
- Ice cream. Instead, choose low-fat cheese, skim milk, or soy milk.
- Roasted nuts. Instead, choose fresh or raw nuts.
- Saturated solid fats or oils. Instead, choose olive oil, sesame oil, canola oil, or flaxseed oil.

Guard Against Benign Prostatic Hyperplasia

Adding the vitamins, minerals, nutrients, and foods listed below to your diet and avoiding alcohol, especially beer, may help to prevent benign prostatic hyperplasia.

The following nutrients may be taken with their respective daily dose:

Zinc 60 mg
Selenium 200 mcg
Vitamin B6 100 to 200 mg/d
Essential fatty acids 1,000 to 2,000 mg
Pumpkin seeds and squash seeds half to one ounce
Saw palmetto, which is an alpha blocker and works like the drug tamsulosin HCl (Flomax) 160 mg

Count Your Calories

Remember to keep these calorie counts in mind:

Foods over four hundred calories, eat one quarter serving or avoid one 6 oz bagel: 400 calories or 1 cup of chickpeas: 500 calories.

Foods under 160 to 200 calories, eat half cup at a time.

1 cup of macaroni: 160 calories
1 cup of corn: 160 calories
1 cup of brown or white rice: 200 calories.

For eighty to one hundred calories, eat maximum one cup.

1 cup of skim milk: 90 calories
1 apple (medium size): 80 to 100 calories
1 pear (large): 80 to 100 calories

1 orange (medium): 80 to 100 calories
1 medium-size banana (not ripe): 80 to 100 calories

For forty to fifty calories, eat one to two cups at a time.

1 cup of cantaloupe: 40 to 50 calories
1 cup of kiwifruit: 40 to 50 calories
1 cup of strawberries: 40 to 50 calories
1 cup of zucchini: 50 calories

For twenty to thirty calories, eat as much as you want.

1 cup of eggplant or squash: 20 to 30 calories
1 cup of sweet yellow, red, or green pepper: 20 to 30 calories
1 cup of spinach: 20 to 30 calories
1 cup of broccoli: 20 to 30 calories
1 cup of cabbage: 20 to 30 calories
1 cup of carrot: 20 to 30 calories

Keep Your Eyes on Your Size

If your BMI (body mass index) is as follows:

Less than 18, eat chickpeas, fava beans, red beans, almonds, nuts, and bagels.
If 18 to 25, then you are okay. Continue the switch to healthy foods.
If 25 to 30, then you are overweight. Lose 5 percent of your weight.
If 30 to 35, then you are obese and should seek help from your doctor.
If 35 to 40, you need medical help *today*.

If it is higher than 40, still young and strong, can't lose weight in the next six months and keeps it, then mostly you need surgery that will ensure weight loss.

If you are athletic with good muscle bulk, BMI doesn't fit you; go to waist-to-hip ratio.

Neck and Back Pains

Cervical spine level disc referred pain (C1-C8)
     C5—pain in the shoulder muscles
     C6—the thumb
     C7 and C8—middle finger
     C8—little finger

Thoracic spine disc referred pain (T1-T12)
     T4—nipple pain
     T10—umbilical area, belly button; it can also come from appendicitis

Lumbar spine area referred pain (L1-L5)
     L3—affects the knee
     L4—medial malleolus
     L5—affects the dorsum of foot, big toe, and second and third toes

Sacral spine area referred pain
     S1—little toe and fourth toe

Eyes
     Legally blind—20/200 or less in the better eye
     Low vision—20/70 to 20/200

Causes:

47 percent cataract (highest)

12 percent glaucoma

10 percent uveitis

8 percent adult macular degeneration

4.8 percent diabetic retinopathy. Retina laser surgery is a cause
   of this type of blindness.

8 percent for other factors

Vascular Retinopathy (No Real Treatment Yet)

We can try rutin; it is a flavonoid. It is a strong antioxidant, which
can reduce bleeding in retinopathy. It strengthens the venous
capillaries and reduces the venous leaks of blood and plasma.
It reduces edema in the legs and retinopathy. It strengthens the
collagen, which gives strength and elasticity of the skin and the
arterial and venous capillaries in particular. It is in buckwheat,
citrus fruits, brown tea, and asparagus.

Use a dose of 50 to 100 mg per day of calcium, magnesium, and
vitamin B complex. Plus antioxidants, vitamins A, C, E; zinc;
lutein; selenium; and omega-3 of 1,000 mg per day or more if
your doctor agrees.

Bilberry, vitamin E, and alpha-lipoic acid may not help vision
but improve the retina health; it decreases bleeding, preventing
further deterioration.

For macular edema in diabetic called cystoids macular edema,
you see foggy as if you are looking through a cup of water.

Ginkgo biloba (the macular edema factor) and probably the only one. I will be glad if there's another over-the-counter medicine and works with minimal problems if used wisely.

You can take 150 mg daily for a month. I suggest taking it uninterrupted at night. Every time you have blurry vision when the far vision becomes unclear and shorter, take 150 mg at night till the edema improves. In my experience, one pill can help for three days and sometimes weeks.

Remember all the above medications except vitamin B, calcium, and magnesium. These can increase blood thinning, so be careful and ask your doctor if you are taking blood thinners like Coumadin. You have to reduce the dose or check it by a blood test.

Dry Eye

Vitamin A, less than 5000 IU per day

Flaxseed can be a good remedy for dry eyes.

The best is frequent, regular washing of the face with warm water then press on lower lid from the medial angle to the lateral angle, you stimulate the tears.

Type 2 Diabetes (Control If You Are on Pills)

Avoid Actos (it gives macular edema) and Avandia (increases heart risk) prescription pills.

To have the best blood sugar next day, check blood sugar before you go to sleep. These doses are for a 180 lb person. If it is less than one hundred, eat a small snack.

For 120 to 140 even 160, you are okay since the finger stick is 10 to 15 percent higher than the big elbow vein we use for the laboratory. Anyhow, don't eat before you sleep.

For 160 to 200, take 250 mg Glucophage or 2.5 Glucotrol. If it is 201 to 250, take 2.5 mg Glucotrol plus 250 mg Glucophage.

If you weigh 105 pounds, take half of these recommended doses, but you can adjust the dose to a higher one if the small dose did not work.

CHAPTER 9

Stress

Stress is a common complaint of a lot of people. the patient will say, Aim under stress these days, and if you ask him what is the problem, he usually avoids a full answer. They don't want anybody to know usually.

Stress, what is it?

Suppose you were walking outside, a dog started attacking you, but he is still far. Your brain will give you two choices: either you fight this dog, if you have a stick or a weapon, or you run as fast as you can. It is called fight or flight. What happens is your adrenaline and cortisone hormones are secreted, more sugar is released to the blood from the liver to use for this acute physical work, your pulse and blood pressure goes up, and your pupils widen. After the dog goes away, you will go back to normal in minutes, but you may develop the posttraumatic stress syndrome for a while.

In case you have a divorce case, you have no way to run. The amount of stress is huge; it is every minute. This one you have no flight, and the fight is long. This means that the adrenaline and cortisone secretion is chronic, and the condition now is the stress, which you can't cope with.

Stress can come from a simple traffic jam, but the worst comes after a death of a dear family member and family-related problems, separation, child custody, as well as financial problems like mortgage or kids' change of residence and schools.

A short acute stress is beneficiary and needed like carrying weights or running a marathon.

It is persistent stress when your genes cannot handle it, since there are some people who can manage the stress, which you have in a short period. These people are genetically programmed to handle acute and chronic stress.

For other type of people who can't handle the stress, distress leads to escape (anxiety) or withdrawal (depression) behavior.

Stress can be sickening. Cortisol increases appetite, which increases weight the worst type, the apple-shape type associated with heart disease. It brings diabetes and low immunity; insomnia follows, work disruption, and, in severe cases, disability.

Who doesn't have stress? They are the newborns, people at their early age, and the brain-dead. What I am trying to say is that stress is part of life. In fact, we need to move better and do better. It is the exaggeration of stress that gives problems.

Stress Hormones

Stress stimulates the brain endocrines. It sends stimuli to a gland called the adrenal gland located above the kidney in the back of the belly. Two hormones are secreted.

The first one is adrenaline. It stimulates the sympathetic autonomic nervous system, which raises the blood pressure and the pulse rate and causes sweating. It opens the pupil for sharper vision (like in insomnia) and opens the lung pipes for better breathing in case you have to fight or run. Adrenaline works for a short time; after the stress goes out, the parasympathetic autonomic system is stimulated. It does the opposite of the sympathetic function like reducing the pulse and blood pressure.

The second type hormones are the cortisol and cortisone. They give sugar as more fuel is needed for the fight or flight; sugar feeds the brain and helps energy for tissues. The cortisone works longer than adrenaline in chronic stress. It is the reason for obesity, hypertension, low immunity, stomach ulcers and poor digestion, and retarded growth in the young. Later it can change mood like being angry at all times—this is the fight—or depression, the flight from the problem.

Stress and Other Diseases

Stress stimulates hormones like cortisone. These hormones can reduce immunity, increase blood pressure, increase appetite, and add weight. It can give weakness and depression.

It can increase cardiovascular diseases. Take aspirin 81 mg even if you are forty years old.

For diabetes, treat as per your doctor's order.

For hypertension and strokes, take ACE inhibitors; it reduces high blood pressure. And for strokes, ask your doctor.

Amenorrhea. The brain reduces it as a nonimportant function for now; it happens sometimes in college students during examinations.

Memory problems and Alzheimer's. Take sage tea, curry in foods, and antioxidants and avoid aluminum-containing drugs.

Impotence. See a genitourinary doctor. The anti-impotence drugs can be used temporarily to avoid augmenting the stress but under a physician's order.

Peptic ulcer disease. Take low-fat cheese, low-fat milk, Tums and Pepcid 20 mg (OTC drugs), or Zantac 150 mg twice a day.

Gastroesophageal reflux for pain in the epigastric area. Get Prilosec (OTC drug) for 20 mg twice a day.

For irritable bowel syndrome, take peppermint and chamomile tea. See a gastroenterologist.

Stress Management

Exercise

It is easier said than done. Somebody who just have a stressful problem will not exercise; he is in bad mood. In a few days, when things calm down and the person realizes the extent of the problem, if he talks to a friend, people usually help. The minute he is in this stage, he has to do something about the stress; one way is exercise. The best exercise for this type of people is to find a friend and go together to a gym; but if the stress is mild, walk, run, jump, swim, walk in the mall—do anything to engage your brain. Instead of cortisone hormone secretion in stress reaction, the brain will give the endorphins called the feel-good hormone. You will change the scene around you; you get busy, and it gives more strength the minute you started thinking about exercise. This means you want a way out of your stress, which is in itself good news. The problem is when you don't try to get out of the stress. Try to stop thinking about what happens. Remember that in some rural areas in the Middle East, people are poor. When they meet each other, they say hi and then they ask, "How is your health?" They never ask how much money you have but say enjoy your life and may God give you the luck. And they will say, "One day above the ground is better than one hundred years under the ground, so get over it. Nobody can stop you from crying. In fact, it is healthy, but crying for good is a disaster."

To do that, get involved with your body and exercise—it relaxes you. The brain increases your physical power; it improves sugar and energy, increases metabolism, improves joints, and increases muscle bulk. In the gym, you meet somebody who is just like you. Talk to someone, help someone, wake up.

Later when things calm down, work around the house. Plant roses, peppermint, sage, thyme, squash, and trim trees.

Have a dog; it stimulates you to walk, even run. You can tell them what you can't tell to anybody else. They are loyal; they keep you busy. They can reduce your blood pressure.

Go out. Walk around the lake and go to the park; nature is beautiful.

The most important part, keep your brain busy. Use it or lose it. Open a little shop, sell things on eBay and play cards with friends. Find a friend who takes things easy, who smiles, jokes, and laughs a lot. Friends can be a help or the opposite.

Married people who are happy can help each other. I know that people get very depressed when they lose their partner; these people need support from their families and friends.

Stand-up comedy—this one is of great help. Watch Jay Leno on CNBC as well as the CBS show *Late Show with David Letterman*; they are good. For movies, go to theaters with somebody.

Visit restaurants or better invite people at home and cook for them. People will invite you too. Stress comes from lack of good friends and lack of friendly relations. Don't isolate yourself. Help people in distress; they will never forget you.

Play music. I play the flute. I have dry eyes. Every time I play the flute, I remember my dad, and I cry. Now I know that my lacrimal glands are working.

Sing alone or with a group; this is the best healing factor.

Look what one of the best Egyptian singers said, "Sing for me softly and slowly. Sing for me, and I will give you my eyes."
Singing is the life of the soul. It heals the stressed and the sick. Sing alone. Sing in the house you live in but softly.

The best way to beat stress is to go to your religious places. You meet people, and you hear what calms you down. Help people and remember that you don't have to have money to help. Work, cook for the homeless, and if you have money, remember that the best thing money is good for is to help people. My god, you feel so good. Help the poor, go work in a soup kitchen. You will know that your problem is nothing compared to others.

Sleep enough hours.
Another way, if you have a few thousand dollars, which you can play with in the stock market, have an account in a stock trade company—and there are a lot of them. Do day or even hour trading. When you start reading about stocks, compare who will go up tomorrow or today. For example, go to Yahoo and see which

companies are going to announce their quarterly income. Study them, see their evaluation. If you feel the stock is good, buy it. After that, protect yourself from large loss.

In the morning, check Yahoo for the most active, the most percentage gain stocks. Read about them. This type of trading is so good that when you win, you feel good; and if you lose, it usually is not a big loss. Your brain was functioning, you stopped thinking about your problems for a while, and no matter what the results were, you had something to brag about or to laugh at your loss. Since not too many make money in the stock market, No gambling here please, and watch Mr. Cramer on CNBC at night you can understand stocks better.

One more thing, don't hurt your children. If they do wrong, just turn your face or avoid them. Let them know you are upset, but they are part of your body, and will you harm yourself?

A Tylenol is okay. Chamomile with green tea, a nerve-soothing tea, is the best.

Chamomile and anise or peppermint does the same.

If you feel or if somebody feels you are suicidal, a psychiatric help is indicated and don't wait.

Remember that stress has something to do with aging and with the five major killers—diabetes, high blood pressure, obesity, high cholesterol, and smo

Chapter 10

Living a Longer, Stronger Life and Looking Good After Forty

Some people say that aging starts after you are born. Let us say it starts after twenty-three, since according to most parameters, you continue your growth up to age twenty-three years.

But forty is a definite switch in your body, and three things happen.

- Small bowel absorption of the food we eat decreases, so even if you eat enough and healthy, you may lack some nutrients.
- Your body metabolism decreases.
- Death or loss of function of very important cells like nerve cells in the brain (from one hundred billion at early life to eighty billion by age fifty) and insulin cells in the pancreas (million at early life to half by age sixty-five, if you did not beat it hard with sweets).

The age switch varies in some people. It may be at thirty-five or less if you have a chronic disease; in others, it may be at age forty-five.

It is my intention to tell you how to increase the life of these dying cells or nonfunctioning cells and to keep your memory and metabolism in good shape.

At forty, you should check for any possible negative factors like high cholesterol, diabetes, overweight, smoking, family history of high blood pressure or heart attacks, and breast cancer or prostate cancer . . . and how to check yourself from a lot of diseases. You should start by visiting your doctor and getting a health profile. Blood, urine, and EKG tests are done to evaluate liver, kidney, and other blood parameters once a year but may be even more if needed; your doctor should decide.

Now to make things better for you, to help you to live with fewer incidences of strokes and to avoid heart attacks, and to make the chronic disease less debilitating, I suggest some old and new ideas mostly known to a lot of people. But I just want to remind you to go back to the proper road in case you have deviated from that road. Eat food you know are good for you rather than what taste good. Exercise; avoid obesity; reduce or stop smoking and drinking alcohol; learn about antioxidants, vitamins, minerals, and trace elements; and lastly fight stress.

Acquired and genetic chronic diseases can be avoided with preventive measures or at least make them bearable.

Getting older, we can't stop that, but don't forget that age is a number. And your physiological age can be younger or older than this number, depending on your genetics, if you are lucky, or if you are smart, knowing how to avoid coming diseases.

To start, we discuss lack of exercise. This is a disease in itself just like poor diet. If you do not exercise and follow a poor diet, you will develop low immunity and chronic inflammations, which are the main cause of early aging and chronic diseases.

In addition to other diseases, which affect you after age forty, are cancer and diabetes.

Since you are not the only alive person in the USA, the government has its problems, so help yourself and don't depend on anyone else. And remember that every seven seconds a baby is born in the USA, and every thirteen seconds someone dies.

Now we can't stop death. But we can make it less painful and less costly. I'd like you to avoid a long stay in the nursing home.

Also, every thirty-one seconds, an immigrant arrives to the USA. The reason is that they want to live better, healthier, and freer.

It is true that we may complain about our health system, but remember, if you go as an emergency case to any American hospital with or without insurance, by law they have to treat you as good as any other person who has insurance; and this may cost large amounts of money. Not too many countries do this.

We can't stop death, but we can prolong your life and try to make you live healthy till the day you die.

I want you to sing till you die.

Now what I am trying to say is that we all will grow old. Being old is beautiful if you are not disabled or in a semicoma state.

It was mentioned that life starts after sixty. In fact, it was found that the best years of your life are from sixty to sixty-nine years if you are healthy.

Accidents happen, and we accept it; but getting a cancer for few years and not knowing about till you go to the hospital as an emergency with a late-stage cancer is not acceptable.

To continue, smoking after a heart attack is insane.

Having a stroke—which came from your carotids and you have multiple episodes of dizziness and temporary blindness for few seconds at a time called transient ischemic attacks of the brain, and sometimes it even gives falls—is not acceptable either because your body had warned that there is something wrong or simply because you never had it before. If you have no contraindication, take a baby aspirin and seek help. Please take care of it; go to your cardiologist or vascular surgeon.

What happened in the past century?

It is lack of exercise. We have to revive the walking we used to do before the cars arrived.

Remember that in 1917, minimal cars were used in the USA. In 1967, there were eighty-nine million cars. In 2006, there were almost three hundred million cars. (i.e., Walking is less and less, so you have to exercise. And I will tell you how.)

In the USA, we are number 42 in life expectancy average compared to the world.

Canadians live two years more, and still they spend half the money we spend per person per year on health care. We spend six thousand dollars; they spend three thousand dollars per year.

There are multireasons for that, and we will discuss it later.

Cancer

A lot of cancer cases have to be controlled better—find it early. It is good for you and your family and to the country. So when it comes to cancer, insist on early detection.

Eating Habits

Donuts, pizza, fast food, white bread, butter, the regular, 64 oz cup of Coke and the extrasize french fries—these are not good for your health. Even if you are healthy, switch now to the farmer's son's diet.

Now . . . exercise. it can be part of your work, like truck drivers, who carry and push heavy objects during the day has ample exercise, but a computer operator person sitting the whole day, or standing as a teacher, then sit on a couch and watch TV at night when he goes home. They represent what we call sedentary life and they have to exercise because exercise can keep their muscles in good tone and strength.

Exercise keeps you adding muscle tissue, and this muscle tissue improves your metabolism. In fact, it keeps the high metabolism hours after exercise, and that will burn the fat or carb. You eat and prevent it from being deposited as fat in the muscles and under the skin.

Exercise is the cheapest way to keep healthy bones, improve diabetes, lose weight, and reduce stress. It increases adrenaline, noradrenaline, serotonin (dopamine)—the pleasure hormone.

Now to keep the energy high, it helps to get carbs, fats, proteins, vitamins, and supplements. The amount of best foods to eat, you will find it in this book.

How Do We Age?

There is something called the free radicals or the oxidants or the reactive oxidants. They are of three types: superoxide, peroxide, and hydroxyl.

These free radicals have to be neutralized or they will attack your cells, mitochondria, and the DNA.

By the way, the major source of free radicals is the mitochondria, the energy factory motors of your cell.

Unneutralized free radicals can damage the bad cholesterol, giving inflammation and vascular blockage.

The worst effect of free radicals is on the brain, resulting to Alzheimer's and chronic brain diseases.

Sources of Free Radicals

Free radicals come from normal energy production in the cell infection, detoxified substances, pollution, cigarette smoking, and exposure to ultraviolet rays by the retina and the skin.

Put it this way: it is the garbage of cell energy end products or outside toxins.

These free radicals can injure the mitochondria, a small area in each cell, which gives energy or life to each cell. Vitamins C and E and other antioxidants can stop that; others like zinc antagonizes it by being part of enzymes that antagonize free radicals.

The cell wall and mitochondria are attacked by these free radicals, weakening them plus reducing their survival, giving chronic diseases like Alzheimer's and parkinsonism.

ABDALLAH TAHA, M.D., F.A.C.S.

The mitochondria has a wall. This wall has small holes. The CoQ10 can enter through it and stimulate or ignite the mitochondria to give ATP and energy. In the process it needs a cardiolipin, which is in the wall of the mitochondria; and it is usually low in the heart, muscles, and brain after forty. It is called carnitine; they are present in foods like meat and also in pills.

Antioxidants

These are taken as pills or fruits and vegetables, beans, or seeds.

Let us start with vitamin A and beta-carotene. Vitamin E and C, selenium, and zinc—all these are found in an over-the-counter pill named Protegra. Take one per day if over fifty and twice a day if you have a negative factor. Ask a doctor if you are taking blood thinners like Coumadin.

It also comes in thousands of chemicals like the flavonoids and phytochemicals. It is in fruits, vegetables, grains, beans, and a lot of other foods.

Healthy Life Helpers

Screening for cancers and using vaccines to avoid infection or cancer and treatment of early diseases and good memory all need some smart habits in eating, exercising, living with minimal stress in addition to some knowledge about what to eat and how to live to make your life less stressful. And when this stress comes against your will, how does your body absorb it without failure?

As a farmer's son, I know they walk and work physically. They eat raw foods and fruits fresh or dried, whole grains, beans, and olive oil. They live in small villages, and they know each other. If someone gets sick, he will have a lot of visitors. Visiting is a must, and it helps stress. Yes, it does help to have friends who care about you.

Now to keep the energy coming and efficient, it helps to get vitamins and supplements especially if you have a chronic Disease.

Vitamins and supplements decrease the free radicals' effects, which is the cause of chronic degenerative diseases like arthritis. Free radicals accelerate aging, shorten the nerve cell life that lead to Alzheimer's and parkinsonism, close vessels, and would result to heart and blood vessel disease.

Free radicals start and increase clotting in the arterial vessels, resulting to poor circulation and gangrene.

Let us start with vitamin A and beta-carotene. Vitamins E and C, selenium, zinc, the flavonoids, and phytochemicals are in fruits, vegetables, grains, beans, and a lot of other foods; these are called the antioxidants.

The maximum amount of antioxidants like in a fixed weight are present in the black and blue berries. They have the highest antioxidants but with high calories. Strawberries have moderate calories. Garlic has minimal calories. Brussels and broccoli and red fresh peppers have low calories. Black and red grapes have moderate calories. This type of grapes gave the French less heart attacks because like red wine; it can improve the heart circulation except that when compared to wine, you can eat more grapes and have less toxicity and accidents.

Probably the most antioxidants we get are from the coffee, tea—especially the green tea—and beans since we eat them daily and in large amounts.

Beans, seeds, and nuts are high in antioxidants but with high calories.

And in this book you will find pomegranate, thyme, and honey; they have more than any of the above.

Antioxidants Value

Antioxidant value is measured by the TAC or total antioxidant capacity and ORAC or oxygen radical absorption capacity.

If you are a diabetic, to improve the quality of life and improve postoperative recovery and improve healing, you have to strengthen immunity and increase cell energy.

Sugar Control

Omega-3: An Anti-inflammatory

Zinc is part of the immunity enzymes. It improves lymphocytes function, replication, and activity. It can decrease HIV progression and can improve immunity in sickly and in alcoholics.

Vitamin C. Its deficiency can decrease immunity and may increase the risk of getting cancer of the lungs and infections. It is present in high concentrations in the red blood cells.

Selenium is an antioxidant.
B-carotene as antioxidant, it decreases risk of cancer of the lungs.
Black seeds paste or crushed seeds

Memory Help

Vitamin B6
Vitamin B12
Zinc
Bea pollen
Folic acid
Omega-3
Rosemary tea (good)
Cardamom add to coffee (good)
Sage with tea (best)
Boron
Garlic
Ginkgo biloba (the French believe it is good)
Antioxidants again are very important
High unsaturated fats like fish, olive oil, walnuts and almond,
    soybean
Increase mental activity
Decrease stress like vacation and stand-up comedy
No alcohol
Stop smoking

Causes for Poor Memory

- Poor nutrition
- Poor brain circulation, check your carotids. Take ginkgo
  biloba; it increases circulation to the brain.

- Alcohol
- Free radicals from toxins like pesticides, lead, ultraviolet rays, and mercury. Eat foods with antioxidants or take vitamin supplements.
- Aluminum
- Statin effect some more than others, and atorvastatin is one of them
- Chronic diseases like hypertension, HIV, and addiction
- Race
- Age over seventy
- Lack of wealth
- Low sugar
- Alzheimer's disease
- Stress

Living Healthy After Forty: Avoiding Disabling Diseases

It is common sense. Most people can survive till age forty even if they are obese or with juvenile diabetes unless they get cancer or real chronic diseases like serious congenital heart or lung problems, which doesn't respond to treatment, and the and the same is true with accidents.

Some people say that aging starts after you are born. Let us say it starts after twenty since according to most parameters you continue to grow up to age twenty-three years in absorption. But forty is a definite switch in your body.

Metabolism. Losing more cells like brain and insulin cells and decrease in absorption from the intestine.

In some it may be thirty-five, in others it may be forty-five. It is our duty to tell you how to increase the life of these dying cells to keep your memory and metabolism in good shape.

At forty, you should check for any possible negative factors: cholesterol; diabetes; overweight and obesity; smoking; family history of high blood pressure, heart attacks, breast cancer, and prostate cancer.

Once a year, you should start to evaluate what you can't check yourself like functions of the liver and kidney and other blood parameters such as cholesterol but may be even more if needed. A doctor should be asked for this test.

By the time I started to think about this book, and now I believe that it is recommended to check yourself at age thirty-five and, in the presence of a family history of diseases, to even start at a younger age. I have seen breast cancer in women in their twenties.

When I say healthy, what does it mean?

Mentally functioning mobile and able—healthy.
Mentally functioning, mobile, but legally disabled—legally blind.
Mentally functioning, immobile, and disabled—hip fracture.
Nonfunctioning, immobile, and disabled—brain-dead or
    vegetable type

After age forty, we will explore how to survive and how to live with good health. So in order to live healthy, we have to start checking ourselves at age thirty-five so we can register the normal values we have. The problem with what I am saying is that some diseases, like type 2 diabetes, starts earlier now than before because of changes in eating and of sedentary habits. Everybody has a car, and walking is minimal now. People at young age, go to the doctor if they feel sick or for vaccines, but after forty, they have to start what we call preventive medicine. check for high cholesterol, diabetes, and hypertension.

Someone Functioning Even with a Problem

- Somebody who can walk or have the ability to reach places even on a wheelchair. His brain is still functioning; he knows what he is doing, where he is going; he can come back if he leaves home, and he can seek help if needed.
- Awake and alert.
- He can see even if he is legally blind with a vision of 20/200 still.
- He can manage to move around. I am not saying that a blind man can't walk or move. I am talking about recent blindness; it is disabling, and it is different from someone who grew up like that. They can manage in a way, and you can't believe how much they can do.
- A person who can hear even with a hearing aid can avoid accidents, which are common in hearing loss. Life is tough on people who are newly deaf, but it is less difficult to live with if it is since childhood. Those who learned the sign language or read lips are in a better situation.
- Smelling and touching are good but not important like the previous cases.
- Eating, even if he has a tube in his stomach and can feed himself, that's okay. I did see a patient who came drunk to the emergency room. The liquor went through his gastrostomy

tube, a tube inserted in his stomach through the skin. Because he has blockage of his food pipe, the man came into the emergency room walking.

Brain Function

- It is to control all central nervous system.
- It is responsible for vision, hearing, taste, olfaction or smell, and all types of coordination between organs.
- It has one hundred billion neurons at young age.
- With all this strength in number and function and sophistication, it can survive for less than five minutes without oxygen.
- It works by receiving signals, process the signals, then react by a reflex or learned experience. Signals will be like the sense of hearing, smell, taste, looking for food, recognizing someone, or muscle movements by using the cortex, cerebellum, and basal ganglia.

Brain Stem

It is the center of automatic function—heart, breathing, locomotion, reflexes, and some hormones, directing the fight, fright, and flight reflexes.

The Mentally Able, Mobile, and Healthy

- They have all the senses normal. They have no chronic disease. They can be a truck driver, a soldier, a personal trainer, or a computer operator.
- They may have some diseases but with minimal effect on their function like prediabetic stage.

- We can call the person healthy and able but limited if he can walk, talk, and think; under no physical stress; he can hear; see better than 20/100; can dress; and can cook, eat, and can carry things.
- He may have conditions like high blood pressure or high cholesterol, a heart stent, leg pain on walking or claudications, or any negative factor with minimal complications yet.

Alive, Healthy But Immobile and Disabled

Examples are fracture hip, spine, and moderate strokes. He is awake, can think, can respond and talk with or without difficulty. He is semihealthy. Although he is a prisoner in his house, he still can eat and ask for help. The minute he can manage to go to the bathroom without exposing his private parts to others, I consider him alive and healthy since he has crossed the red lines. He can do standing and little walking.

The Vegetative State

Just like the alive type or nonfunctioning and disabled, those who are alive but mentally can't respond like Ms. Schiavo's case. If you remember her case, sometimes we call them no code patients, which means doctors do not resuscitate them if they develop cardiac arrest. If the family agreed, and that happened to my own brother, it means there is no hope that the patient will ever recover. Their electroencephalogram will give a brain-dead type print.

Since their brain test showed no activity or brain-dead, this type is the sad type. Ms. Schiavo's case came from very low potassium after taking water pills for a heart condition. The treatment is a few dollars a day and a blood test to check for the potassium level. The doctor has to order this test for this type of patients. If the patient doesn't agree, he should be removed from the doctor's practice. If the doctor failed to ask for this cheap test, he will pay later in a sue case in millions.

Now to explain it more, a diabetic can lose both legs, can be on dialysis, and can survive a heart attack; but still he can have a conversation with the ambulance driver, can go to his doctor in a wheelchair, can complain and thank his health professional. I mean he is still alive and can survive with the help of another man without any heart disease, with functioning lungs and kidneys. But patients with stroke, the hemiplegic type, the brain is poorly working. He can't void or move his bowels or even answer well.

That's the sad type; please avoid it. Avoid strokes by taking aspirin, statins, ACE inhibitors, even vitamin E and antioxidants. If you can't take other meds, insist on something from your doctor. Operations or any other way, we will mention.

All that I want to do is keep you at least alive and functioning and even mobile, but don't forget that mobility without a brain is not good, as in Alzheimer's type 1 and type 3.

What Are the Common Disabling Diseases?

Strokes

Most of my family elders died from stroke while in good health and walking. A three cent per pill of baby aspirin could have changed that, at least to change the stroke from fatal in one day to a small one, which you can recover from. I am saying that because at their time they did not know about carotid operations in that area.

That's why I suggest a law to do an ultrasound test on both carotids, abdominal aorta, and legs to rule out a threatening vascular disease; otherwise we will keep getting the problems which is costly at a personal, family, and work levels. To be sure that what happened to my family years ago would not happen to America, the wealthy, live with simple measures to keep the brain healthy.

It can be prevented or its injury reduced. Yes, on high number of cases, and that case can be yours.

Ninety percent of strokes can be controlled.

Strokes are of three types:

- Occlusion of specific brain vessel by a clot or embolus from the heart or carotids. These are preventable; these are over 90 percent of strokes.
- By bleeding in or around those vessels. It is a bad case.
- Less common other causes are tumors.

Since 90 percent of strokes come from hard emboli from the carotids and to a lesser extent from soft emboli from the heart, these emboli or small solid calcium or small soft blood spheres can be stopped. And even if you get it, you have seventy-five to ninety minutes to clear it or reduce its danger so that you can live with it. This happens if you go to the proper hospital initially and not by transferring from one hospital to another.

So What Can We Do for This Problem?

Doctors should check carotids for murmurs. If you are over fifty and your doctor doesn't check your carotids when you visit him even for a cold, see another doctor. If you have no murmurs, a baby aspirin is good. If you have carotid murmurs, a Doppler ultrasound of the carotid is needed; and later, you may need carotid angiogram if the ultrasound is positive.

Even magnetic resonance imaging (MRI) or magnetic resonance angiography (MRA) will tell them medical or surgical treatment is done, the complications are low, and the results are astonishing. I was there.

For abdominal aortic aneurysm, computed tomography (CT) scan or ultrasound is suggested. A large murmur is heard if you have this aneurysm in the belly. This type of aneurysm, if more than five centimeters should be repaired if indicated. If it ruptures while you are at home, you have 10 percent chance to survive even with operation. Because the bleeding is so massive, most of the blood will be around the aorta and in the belly. The death is usually from shock from the blood loss. Imagine an artery of three to five and sometimes ten centimeters is ruptured and is bleeding. It is a disaster. A hundred-dollar ultrasound can catch it.

I heard an advertisement that an ultrasound technician's father died from a similar condition. Now he has at home an ultrasound to check the carotid, aorta, and legs for a low fee because he doesn't want anybody at old age to die from these well-conquered diseases, so his father can be proud of him. I salute him. All states should have someone him. It should be done every few years.

If you do it early, you may have complications in a low percentage, but death is very low. If you have an abdominal aortic aneurysm (AAA), do it. Treatment has changed these days to a less invasive type.

It appears that each country or adjacent countries has different factors to extend life and avoid health disasters. In Japan, they eat soybeans; they also don't develop breast cancer. In Okinawa, they eat coral calcium, which is a raw type from the sea and has up to sixty other additional nutrients. In fact, they eat up to 15 g calcium a day. We eat one and a half grams daily. Usually, your calcium has nothing else with it, so don't take more since I call it the processed calcium. For calcium to be used by the body, it needs copper, magnesium, manganese, zinc, and a lot of factors, which are present in coral calcium and not in the calcium pills.

The islanders, they eat the cold seawater fish, which is high in omega-3 and low in toxins. They live long even when they are overweight.

The French Paradox

The French eat high fat food like the Americans, but they live longer and with less heart attacks; they drink wine or eat black grapes and more beans. It is the red and black grapes that has the coronary dilator resveratrol, and that made the difference.

In the Mediterranean area, they eat fat meat but once or twice a week and use olive oil daily and grapes, other fruits, and vegetables. They live long; it is the olive oil here that is the life extender.

These things may sound simple, but it is not.

Those foods I mentioned are eaten daily, but I am sure about something else. All the people I mentioned move around or at work more than we know. They fish with a small boat, rowing. This is exercise, and they smell the best air in that sea.

In these days, most of us here drink soft drinks with the high-fructose corn syrup, eat in the fast-food restaurants since we have cars. And in most cases in these countries, things have changed to the worse. By the way, even the countries I mentioned with less heart diseases are now eating our food; they want to feel rich probably.

How about Us Here?

The American diet is a high-carb, high-protein, high-fat diet. It is the rich-country diet. I say that since the rich people in this country are less obese than the poor and middle class and since everybody can eat their meals a day, even the poor. This type of diet—high-carb, high-fat diet—results to obesity, diabetes, and hypertension. And if you smoke and with a family history of certain diseases, you add more risks.

To change what we eat may take a long time. These things are built in the culture. Some people live like they are in Halloween all the time.

In a village in Italy, people were overweight but lived long; they were found to eat more olive oil. I am talking about olive oil in salads, alone with bread, and used in cooking, so they are eating it a few times a day. And that's why it makes a difference—it reduces the cholesterol.

In India they eat curry. I mean a lot of it. If you pass in front of their houses, you will smell it. They have minimal cases of Alzheimer's disease. Eating only what they eat is fine, what is not mentioned in the books is that these people live in mountainous areas or near the sea and may not have cars. They plant, they cut trees, and they carry products even at old age. I saw a guy on TV age eighty-five. In a little boat, fishing, he dives to position the fishing net. That even is as important as eating the fish. Know that it is suggested that we take more omega-3 and less fish because the lake-type fish has toxins.

So it is the whole situation, not the food alone.

So far, wine in small amounts or black grapes, olive oil, omega-3, cold-sea fish, fruits, and vegetables can help you survive in a better health.

Coral Calcium, Soybeans Give a Difference, So Try Them

So far we can't stop some cancers, but we can find them early and decrease their problems.

We can't stop trauma like car accidents, but we can make them less in number and severity.

We can't stop psychosis, but we can make it more manageable.

Also, we can prevent a lot of disabling diseases. The problem in disabling diseases is that it is tough to remove from the dictionary. So we have to deal with it.

Strokes: It Is a Real Disaster and in High Percentage But Can Be Avoided and Prevented

Ninety percent of strokes come from the heart and carotids, but the carotids are much more in incidence.

The carotids are two in number. They run adjacent to the air pipe. If you compress them, you can stop high percentage of the blood going to the brains and pass out. In some people, they are so sensitive that if the shirt collar presses even mildly, the person may feel like passing out. And if he doesn't loosen the collar, he may pass out. The reason is the condition called vasovagal syncope, which is secondary to stimulation of the tenth cranial nerve, giving a low heart rate like forty beats per minute. Usually, it is sixty to ninety beats per minute. With low pulse, the brain can't get enough blood. After falling and lying down, the flat position relieves it. Staying few minutes flat or with legs up, it will take care of the problem. Just be sure you have no injury from the fall.

The carotids can narrow with age, especially at the bifurcation. In the middle of the neck in the front, this condition is one of the most conquered diseases, which, if not treated, may give an embolus in the brain that can destroy your life and the people you love since that's how it gives the stroke.

If you are over fifty and with any negative factor like high blood pressure, diabetes, or vascular disease and your doctor doesn't put his stethoscope on the middle of your neck to check your carotids, don't go back to him because he treats diseases and does not prevent diseases. A murmur can be detected, and a noninvasive carotid test can be done. The narrowing can be judged as minor or severe. Blockage needs an operation after an arteriogram, and less than that, it can be treated with blood-thinning medications, but remember each case is different and what fits may be different. For example, they may find one carotid is closed already, now the other has to be dealt with, and it is a problem. By the way, it took years before you reach this stage, and most of the time you get something called transient ischemic attacks. The stroke comes from a detached piece of the blocking plaque. If the plaque is small, it will be carried with the blood to the brain on the same side. It will give you the transient ischemic attack, which is a temporary loss of vision on that side, loss of balance, and dizziness. Take two baby aspirins and go to the emergency room in a big hospital. Don't take just lying down.

If the detached plaque is more than 3 mm, it will give the stroke, which is characterized by loss of function on one side of the face and the arm and leg on the other side. You have to go to a stroke center; otherwise, go to a trauma-type center. Don't go to a small hospital unless it is the only hospital in the area. The reason for that is that you have certain amount of time for testing and treatment. And at night and even in the daytime in some hospitals, you will be delayed because of lack of machines and specialists, so tell your family where to go if something big happens.

Strokes are disabling. In addition of loss of a lot of functions, it can give decubitus ulcers and pulmonary and leg emboli. And it is costly.

The noncarotid cause of stroke is 10 percent. It can be from bleeding, rupture from aneurysm, which is a small thin dilatation of a small vessel in the brain, trauma and bleeding, and thrombosis of a vessel.

All these are difficult to control if it happens, but you have to know that except for trauma, most of the time there are some signs, which precede these disasters, like recurrent headache, sometimes severe one-sided weakness, unexplained with temporary vision loss and dizziness. These may be an indication of that aneurysm. Usually there are symptoms. Go to a neurologist, cardiologist, and neurosurgeon for headaches. Be aggressive; it is your good life on the line.

Aneurysms in small vessels can be diagnosed and clipped by a neurosurgeon.

Bleeding sometimes can come from blood thinning overdose; you have to check your blood thinning level with your doctor frequently since overdose is as bad as low dose.

So in addition to strokes, what are those other diseases which can put you in a disabling condition? Some are less disabling than others but most are. Avoid if you can.

Bones—fracture of the hip and fracture of the spine. Avoid osteoporosis. These are the second worst disabling condition after strokes. They can kill by giving pulmonary emboli, which come mainly due to immobility. Remember here DEXA scan and calcium intake.

Alzheimer's disease. Remember President Reagan. See what you can do not to get Alzheimer's. It is crippling to the person and the family. Imagine you can't open a door in the house and keep it open since the patient can leave and not come back because he reversed to child brain size.

Late-stage cancers. Avoid this disaster by checking yourself early. If you feel change of bowel habits, bleeding even small from the mouth, urethra, rectum, or vagina at old age, better check it now. At every age level, you should check for most common tumors. Like doing colonoscopy at age fifty, don't forget anticancer vaccines or a blood test for prostate cancer at age fifty-two in men and a Pap smear in women.

Acute heart attacks or unexpected arrhythmias. Avoid cardiac myopathies and heart muscle hypertrophy. See a heart doctor once even if your internist refuses that.

Medication errors, allergy, or interactions with anaphylactic reaction. Read the labels of Penicillin and Avalox in particular.

Coma. Avoid brain injuries, brain bleeding from meds like strong blood thinners. Read the pharmacy information given to you when you pick up your medicine, or let somebody read it for you. Ask your doctor, especially if you are taking Coumadin or Plavix given to avoid strokes and heart attacks.

Infections like HIV, polio, plaque, and infectious diseases. Get the vaccines like measles, mumps, and rubella if you are born before 1958.

Pulmonary emboli come from deep venous thrombosis of the legs or pelvic veins. If it is not deadly, it is crippling. Good measures can decrease it including inferior vena cava filter. Doctors have to be aggressive here.

Blindness. Take care of your diabetes. For bad eye disease, go to institutions and not simple doctors.

Treat brain tumors and abnormal movement like chorea and parkinsonism. Avoid falls. Protect the hip area with a special protector.

Control chronic diseases like diabetes, heart conditions, high blood pressure, and sleep disorders, which can give abnormal heart rhythm and heart attacks.

What Are the Common Functions That Make You Disable?

- Can't feed self.
- Can't move and can't pass urine in the bathroom or move bowels independently.
- Can't clean after bowel movements.
- Can't grab things you need.
- Poor or no mental function. This is the worst, it is the vegetative state.

How to Reduce Disabling Diseases?

What can we do to reduce these problems?

- Aspirin, a baby aspirin or larger dose, according to condition. Plavix is another medicine and sometimes both. It can reduce heart attacks and strokes.
- Exercise done right according to age and health. It has no equal in all mentioned remedies.
- Doctors should check for carotid murmurs, at least after age forty, and ultrasound of carotids after fifty or if indicated at any age to see if there is any plaques. If the carotid has 90 percent occlusion or is symptomatic like it gave a small stroke or transient ischemic attack in which you have a temporary loss of vision or consciousness, you may need an operation which removes the plaques. It is lifesaving.
- Check eyes. Improve vision to avoid falls and accidents.
- Avoid falls and strenuous exercises.
- Vaccines, according to age, stop meningitis and pneumonia and cancers in females.
- Cancer checkup. Don't come with a late-stage cancer. The most frequent in females is the breast cancer and in the males is the prostate. And both can be caught early and treated nicely. Don't wait to investigate these tumors; it is a must if you have a family history.
- Diet. Eat well, drink spring water and eat fruits. Vegetables, nuts, beans with low glycemic load. Fish once or twice a week. Meat twice a week, dairy products, low fat and olive oil, some spices, some supplements, if needed. Some

antioxidants antagonize cancer. Some vitamins are anticancer. High fiber can reduce colon cancer.

- Check for diseases like HIV if you have a reason. HIV positive is not AIDS. AIDS comes after five to ten years after the infection. HIV patients can live more than diabetics if they get treated.
- If you travel outside the USA, take prophylactic vaccines or antibiotics from your doctor.
- Anti-inflammatory. The new thinking is that inflammation of the vessels are very important because of aging and most of the chronic diseases. Aspirin is an anti-inflammatory drug.
- In fact, anticholesterol meds may work by its anti-inflammatory action on the vessels. The inflammation is caused by the free radicals, which blocks the small as well as the large vessels that will cut off the oxygen and food to the cells, giving them ischemia and short life. The antioxidants, anticholesterol meds, and aspirin all antagonize these free radicals.
- Don't go to a doctor who is your family friend since the exam will be deficient.
- Review the poly pill and ask your doctor.
- Vitamins, antioxidants, and minerals.
- Weight loss if overweight.
- Laugh, work, and use it or lose it. Keep your brain functioning.
- To decrease acute disabling infections, do not forget the vaccines.

Adult Vaccinations

It depends on health, age, previous immunizations, lifestyle, and travel location.

Varicella

Ninety-seven percent of population are immune. Getting the disease at young age gives you immunization forever. If you are not sure about the disease and the vaccinations, you can take the antibody titer test. If you are not immune, you better have one, especially if you are in the patient care business. This is a live virus, not given in low-immunity cases like AIDS patients.

Hepatitis A

To those travelling to Central and South America, check for other countries' people who have liver disease. It is given in two separate doses.

Hepatitis B

- Travelers and health professionals'. You need three doses over four months' period.
- Flue shot.
- To people over sixty-five or at any age if they have negative factors. Some suggest over fifty. Some factories give it yearly to its employees to reduce off days due to the virus.
- MMR for adults born after 1958. It is a live virus, so no patient in pregnancy, nursing, or low-immunity is advised. This is good for twenty years.

Polio

Just to those who are travelling to certain areas.

Tetanus/Diphtheria

Its immunity goes for ten years. Adults are advised to get it. It is a deadly virus with little reactions.

Pneumococcal vaccine for people at risk for pneumococcal pneumonia and meningitis.

More than sixty-five years old or above two years with chronic diseases like heart failure, cirrhosis, asplenism, sickle cell, diabetes mellitus, immune suppressed, leukemia. Good for five to ten years.

Screening for Cancer

The American Cancer Society said, "Believe it; we have six thousand less deaths in 2004 than in 2003."

But still it is high. We have over half million deaths per year, and don't forget, every new year we have more aging population, and that makes the news even better. This doesn't include around one million cases of different skin cancers since mostly, it is not deadly except for melanoma.

The main reason of lowering the death rate is better screening 33 percent of cancers. It can be prevented if we screen people right with change of lifestyle, proper diet and self exam, more activity, and smoking cessation. When you catch cancer early, mostly you will not need radiation or chemotherapy.

There is a lack of funding for some cancer research, and million Americans are smoking, and 90 percent of those who develop lung cancer are chronic smokers.

The cancer screening is avoided sometimes because of lack of funds, low income, and lack of insurance. Testing is not cheap for a poor or middle-class person.

In the case of smokers, they need help to quit smoking and have a regular screening.

Colorectal Cancer

It is one of the most alleged failures to diagnose. It surpassed the breast cancer or at least equal to it in number.

Most of the doctors sued are the internists and others to a less degree are the gastroenterologists, radiologists, and surgeons.

It is now suggested to have a colonoscopy by age fifty. The problem is that there are cases as young as twenty, so, doctors, better listen to the patient and investigate their symptoms. And to the young patients who have any rectal bleeding at any age, better know the cause and ask for the family history.

How We Do the Screening?

- Rectal exam yearly. After forty and at any age with symptoms.
- Guaiac test. Three specimens of stool, in different days, are checked for blood. If it is done yearly, it can decrease delayed

diagnosis to 33 percent. This test can be bought and done at home but better in the lab.

- Sigmoidoscopy in office procedure. It checks the reason for bright or brown blood. Sixty-seven percent of colorectal cancers are in the last twenty to thirty centimeter of the colon. Sigmoidoscopy cuts down on delayed diagnosis to 67 percent.
- Colonoscopy needs a special operating room or an outpatient surgical center. This is the better test in which the whole colon is inspected.
- Barium enema. It was done more before. Now colonoscopy is done more since a biopsy can be done at the same time.
- CAT scan is good for screening and to rule out other pathology. It can show the degree of metastasis, so really it is done if the patient refuses colonoscopy. Or it is complementary to check the liver and other abdominal contents to know the extent of the tumor.
- Bone scan is to rule out bone metastasis in advanced or suspicious cases.
- Another important factor is the communication between the primary doctor and the patient to keep the schedule of examinations and the radiologist to give accurate and timely results and the gastroenterologist to follow up on the results of colonoscopy and possible surgery. Failure of any step can give the delay in treatment.

Tests Done in the Office

PSA tests are good tests for screening.

- Pap smear is very accurate for cervical cancer or younger if with family history.
- CEA blood test for cancer.

- AFT blood test for liver cancer.
- Guaiac test for occult blood in stool.

The colorectal cancer as well as other cancers' symptoms may be silent. It may take a while before it gives significant bleeding or blockage or pain. It depends on the type of pathology since any cancer has multiple types, and they differ in their speed of growth to be symptomatic and give complications as blockage or as metastasis in the liver, lungs, and bones.

It is common to find polyps on routine colonoscopy, and a high incidence of tumors is in that polyp now or it will change to cancer later in some cases. Finding it early is a blessing. Removal of this polyp is a plus even if it is cancer since it is an early cancer. But the family history, change in bowel habits, like persistent constipation followed by diarrhea, black stool or bloody stools, weight loss, and persistent pain on lower middle back should not be missed. Patient has to be worked up.

I have operated on most of my patients referred in a late stage of cancer, but when people go to a screening colonoscopy, it is now suggested after fifty. Their tumor usually is a small polyp and localized.

If workup after the polyp removal show noninvasive or minimally invasive tumor, it is different from a patient with obstructed colon admitted as an emergency. I never saw an obstructing tumor less than third stage. Which means it involves lymph nodes and penetrated the colon already. Life expectancy will depend on few factors. The most important is the stage of tumors and the pathological type if it is aggressive or not.

For Breast Cancers

A mammogram is good. We start at age forty.

Other modalities like ultrasounds and MRI can help. There is a five-year survival in breast cancer in 75 percent of cases.

Other Cancers

- Gastroscopy for food pipe and stomach cancer is very good.
- Liver. Primary liver cancer is discovered by chance or late in the game.
- Pancreas. This one is usually discovered late with poor prognosis.
- Testical tumors. This is usually missed. Patient should report swelling and changes in size or consistency early and rather be safe than sorry.
- Ovaries. A common type of cancer but with good prognosis. Visit your ob-gyn yearly.
- Skin. Check yourself. You have to ask your doctor about any lump in your body, new or old. Do HPV test and use vaccine before sex starts to stop the cervical cancer.
- Do not laugh at these statistics because a lot of those statistics are people who thought they will never get cancer. Cancer kills more children than any other disease these days.

The most common cancers are the following:

- Lung cancer. It kills 160,000 people per year. Mostly are smokers, so all smokers should be screened by a chest x-ray or better a CT scan. Also there are 213,000 new cases per year.

- Colorectal cancer. Check for stool in blood and colonoscopy after fifty. This is high with family history. It kills 52,000 cases per year with new 112,000 cases per year.
- Breast cancer. A mammogram is done usually after forty but can be done before that as suggested by your doctor. It kills 40,000 cases per year with 150,000 new cases discovered per year.
- Prostate cancer. It kills 27,000 per year with 218,000 new cases. A rectal exam, PSA test, and more specific tests if the condition requires that.

Did you realize that lung cancer kills more people per year than the breast, prostate, and colorectal cancers combined? And listen, these three cancers give three times the number of new cancers per year, which means if you get lung cancer, say by,

And since smoking is the reason in 90 percent of the cases, do you still want to smoke after today?

If you analyze the results, like if somebody told you, you are going to get a cancer. Which one would you choose?

To have prostate cancer, it is slow growing. For each new two hundred thousand cases per year, twenty-seven thousand die. The ratio is one to eight.

In the breast cases, it is around one to four in death per year.
In the colorectal cancer, it is one for each two diagnosed. Lung cancer is the worst, and sometimes it kills in months after diagnosis, so it is the most aggressive.
The worst will be the lung again—it is 1 to 1.5.

DIET

I am a surgeon. I find that most diets came from nondoctors and some cardiologists. Each thinks that his diet is good for anybody.

Well, I don't think so. A diabetic, who is building houses with no other negative factors, is different from his diabetic brother of the same measurements but works as a teacher with no exercise.

Diet should be adjusted according to these factors:

- If you have high cholesterol
- Inactivity
- High blood pressure
- Age after forty
- And even wealth level

Things are not simple, but each one should know some information about his disease level, and the red lines he should not cross.

A brain surgeon knows a lot about the brain, spine, and nerves.

A thoracic surgeon knows about heart and lung surgery.

A general surgeon knows a lot about thyroids, parathyroid, skin tumors, all abdominal problems, from the stomach to the rectum. Usually he knows what vascular problems are; he knows enough medicine that if the internist didn't show up or in an emergency, he can manage till he can get help. Not too many specialties can do that.

Surgeons can put intravenous injections in shocked patients and can treat collapsed lungs like chest surgeons; they can open the chest in a stab wound and can control the bleeding of the heart.

Just put it in your mind that they can manage surgical and internal medicine in any emergency period.

So probably they have some information about a lot of the body emergencies. And if someone can deal with that, I am sure he can do a good job on chronic health problems.

Last thing about surgeons. While they are in residency or in practice, all subspecialties ask them to assist on their operations, so they are aware of what is happening with the other subspecialties like orthopedics, neurosurgery, genitourinary, or thoracic surgery. In fact, we know how much each of these doctors can do. We can deal with any surgical emergency.

Is Your Weight and Shape a Factor in Healthy Life?

Different Shapes of People:

Hourglass
Balloon type (not good)
Apple type (not good)
Thin like a thread
Pearlike

BMI or Body Mass Index: Some Information

BMI mostly tells your type of weight but with some exceptions.

Some has a high BMI but are athletes, so BMI doesn't mean much to them like wrestlers or boxers. It is the relation between your weight in kilogram and your size in meters squared.

Also, the frame of size. Some people are small others are medium or large frames. So you take this into consideration.

Also, some insurance companies warn people to be few pounds extra in case you get sick and without food for few days. Since the amount of intravenous sugar is not enough per day, you have some fat to burn.

It is now suggested to put half to one pound extra per year if you are above sixty years.

BMI is not a part of religion; you keep checking it every day unless you are a fashion model. In fact, I want few pounds extra; in case you fall, fat is a cushion. It can be a fracture protector, or in case you get sick, it is like money in the bank. Your body can use it if you put nothing by mouth.

There are some conditions, which you can live with it, like mild overweight, but obesity is a different category. It can give you or increase your incidence of all bad, disabling problems, the same with other negative factors. It can give a difficult life, and it is painful for you and the family. If you have Alzheimer's, fractured hip in the nursing home, or a stroke and in a semicoma state. What is good about it?

As a surgeon, I believe in case you have obesity and you are with a BMI over forty trying to lose weight for few years and is not working and you are medically eligible for an operation, do it while you are at this stage. Waiting till you have complications like heart and lung problems is not on your side. Do the operation after clearance. There are few of them; find the good hospital before the good doctor.

Age Factor

A simple hernia done on a healthy twenty- to forty-year-old person is done as an outpatient procedure.

But if he is sixty-five, even healthy, we may keep him in the hospital overnight to avoid urine retention and to be sure he goes home with no fever and any lung problem. In fact, we put him on heart monitor during the night but in a regular floor.

This is the age factor only.

But if the patient has diabetes, heart disease, and incarcerated hernia, that makes the problem even more demanding.

Now if this patient comes in with obstructed hernia, with fever, and if usually gangrenous bowel is found in this emergency operation, it may go to a different direction. The incision will be larger or different, and the hospital stay will take longer because he is not fed immediately after small bowel surgery.

The patient who has a piece of intestine removed has to pass gas before eating. It may take days and has to stay in the hospital to be monitored for a leak may happen. A second operation is needed. All these things can happen at any age.

So if you have an hernia anywhere in your body, check with a surgeon and see if it needs repair; do it before it blocks and it goes gangrenous, transforming a simple procedure to a complicated one.

Eye Diseases

It is funny that in this country, you can have a kidney transplant and then live happily.

You can have breast cancer or thyroid cancer or acute chest pain, and after operations, you will do all right in most cases.

But if you get an eye disease or cancer of the lungs or the pancreas within few years, mostly you are disabled or out of good shape.

In the eyes, eye doctors can fix your cataract. It works well.

Also they are successful in correcting refractory vision by the use of laser. By the way, the refractory laser is not a real laser. I am talking about the cornea-type laser. It is some sort of light.

But when the eye doctors go behind the eye lens, they get lost there when they use the laser, as if they are walking in the jungle.

Bone doctors can fix your hip or give you total knee replacement after a good workup.

While other doctors may not do a chest x-ray for a twenty-five-year-old smoker although I'd like to do even a CAT scan on those chronic smokers to catch his cancer early—can anybody tell me why the cancer society asks for a colonoscopy if you are over fifty, but not for a fifty-dollar chest x-ray if you are a chronic smoker? They never advised that yet.

Believe it or not, I came to this country in 1972. The meds for type 2 diabetes did not change that much since then till after the nineties. And even those new drugs are not that better.

While AIDS, which started in the eighties, has so many good meds that I can say that HIV is semiconquered. You can give a pregnant woman one pill and deliver the baby by caesarian; this baby will not develop AIDS. Go figure. Also, an AIDS patient can live longer than diabetics, and diabetes is known for hundreds of years.

Obesity and Surgery

Now the road is as important as the car. So pick a good surgeon; he is important but the equally important is the hospital.

The American College of Surgeons has classified the hospital bariatric operating rooms. Go to the high-star ones. You should go to a good one.

One example why they consider the operating room is good is if they have more than two surgeons who can do this type of operation. This is important for assistance, follow-up, and coverage in case your surgeon is out of town.

Back Injury and Fractured Spine

We can't stop trauma, but we can diagnose osteoporosis and treat it. We can avoid falls; put a helmet if you decide to ride a bicycle. Don't walk into rough areas; check your vision.

No strenuous exercises. You have to know which doctor can take care of you and which hospital to go to. Have your meds written and in your pocket at all times. To check the pressure, make sure to keep the tube of the machine in the middle of the arm, one inch above the elbow, while you are seated and relaxed.

If you want to know if the hospital is fair, just ask if they have obstetrics. Hospitals without delivery services may not have anesthesia at night, and that is dangerous. Remember, when you are very sick or injured, the letters are *a, b,* and *c.* It means airway, breathing, and circulation.

It means if you can't breath, nothing else matters.

The best one and the safest to intubate you to deliver oxygen is an anesthesiologist. Trauma centers will have them at all times. Hospitals with obstetrics have them all the time usually.

Now for a stomach, intestine, hernia, and appendix, most hospital operating rooms can do the job. Even fracture of the hip, you have time to be stabilized or transferred. But not when your life is in danger.

Where to Live?

To be healthy, you have to know where to live: an area with less pollution and better medical facilities.

If you have to live in an area near busy streets, try to avoid the lower floors. Take the highest. If you can travel, find a rural area with trees or running rivers or a sea nearby.

As we said, live in mountains in the middle or the top, far from the streets.

How Can You Check Yourself?

It is simple to check weight, height, and get BMI from the chart. Take into consideration your frame type: small, medium, or large.

If you develop hoarseness of voice for no apparent infection or if it is not going away in one or two weeks, vocal cord tumor has to be ruled out by a throat specialist.

Check mouth for lumps, ulcers, or sores if it doesn't go away in one to two weeks.

Check stool if it is black or mixed with blood.

You may have bleeding; we call it high in origin. Like from the stomach, the iron in the blood cells has time to be digested to the color black. Some meds can do the same like if you are taking iron pills, but if the blood is red, it is from the colorectal area. Other colors can depend on the amount and origin. Blood in the stool or black stool is important and dangerous till it is proven otherwise. Cancer has to be ruled out although other causes may be the reason like bleeding hemorrhoids or diverticulosis of the colon.

If you develop constipation, new or change of bowel habits, including diarrhea, check with a doctor.

So you have a family history.

History of Polyps

Blood in the sputum is an indication of a disease. It may be simple like bronchitis but can also be tuberculosis or cancer. CT scan of the lungs and neck may be needed. I chest pain or chronic bloody greenish sputum

Blood in Urine

It is very important. It can be an infection or stones, but it can be cancer of the bladder or kidney.

Breast lumps, thickening under the skin, bleeding from the nipple, lump in the axilla or armpit, and change in color to red with or without pain.

Vaginal bleeding or chronic bloody discharge less than forty years old, bleeding between menstrual cycles, or excessive bleeding.

Postmenopausal bleeding is cancer unless proven otherwise, and I don't mine if you got scared after reading this.

Testis

Check for a lump and increase in size.

Check Your Feet

The foot has forty-two bones. If they are aligned well, you can walk, run, and jump. If you can't, see a podiatrist. A foot problem can affect your knees and even hips and back.

Medical doctors do not check breasts for tumors; it looks like some patients do not even accept it. Just like surgeons, they do not get involve in heart disease. I am talking about prevention or diagnosis, so it is good to know where to go for each problem.

If you have weight problems and if you are above thirty, fix it. Weight loss is needed.

Blood Pressure Checkup

Buy a blood pressure automatic machine. If you are on meds, check your pressure daily at the same time, few hours after you start your meds. Write it down and show it to your doctor and let him decide and see what he says.

Check your pressure once a week or every few days, same time, same parameters. Like food and rest.

How to Read the Blood Pressure Results?

- First I found that these machines are very sensitive, so few points extra are common.
- Check it at least twice and move the tube more to the inner part of the arm.
- We call the pressure normal if the top one or the systolic is less than 120.
- It is hypertension if it is over 140. Prehypertension is 120 to 129 over 80 to 89.
- It is really the direction of the blood pressure numbers which is important. Like if you take the blood pressure, let us call it BP; and if it is rising monthly, then you start with weight loss. If you are overweight, one point down per one pound loss is possible. Then follow a high-potassium, calcium, and low-sodium diet.

The sodium will keep more water in the circulatory system, increasing the blood volume, and that increases the blood pressure to decrease salt intake. Watch what you eat. No salty cheese, no pickles, no salty peanuts, salty soups in restaurants, and avoid pretzels; but you can eat regular low-fat cheese and unsalted peanuts. Reduce caffeine dose.

Coffee can give temporary high blood pressure, but if you drink six cups a day, that will give you a continuous high BP. At least reduce the number and the size of the cup.

Take tea, the green one. It has caffeine but one-fifth of the amount, and it has other multifactors which can reduce your BP.

Laugh, take vacations, go out, reduce cholesterol—all can help.

A BP of 130 over 90 is the maximum normal.

A checkup is needed, electrocardiogram, liver and kidney test. Blood sugar and cholesterol with anti-inflammatory tests like reactive protein as well as urine test, especially for microalbuminemia. Young people have to be worked up for renovascular disease and even tumors if there is a reason to suspect it.

The same machine will show you the pulse.

You can take advantage of knowing the normal. Again, you check this when you are at rest, physically and mentally. Any physical exercise will increase the pulse; the normal results are between sixty and ninety. A pulse above one hundred at rest has to be investigated. Hyperthyroidism is one reason, and cardiac disease is another.

Pulse over 125 to 170 is a heart conduction sickness and has to be treated.

There are a few heart problems that can give high heart rate like fistulae or a hole between the ventricles, which pumps the blood to the system.

If you are with a fifty-five pulse and you are a very active person, like a marathon runner, it is good. But if you are obese and not very active with low pulse, it is important to see a cardiologist. I've read recently that Mr. Bush has a pulse of forty-five. And that was the reason given when he fell off the couch and sustained a face injury since sometimes people of this low pulse can have dizziness if they stand up suddenly. Treatment is to lie down flat and raise legs up for few minutes. Some may need a pacemaker.

This low pulse can happen in people with normal pulse during blood drawing. The prick gives a low pulse in the forties, and the patient passes out, and it is called vasovagal syncope. It is from the pain of the needle prick. Taking the blood while lying down stops the reaction.

It can also come from pressure on carotids or from severe scary scenes.

Low pulse can come from meds like beta-blockers, so if your pulse goes below sixty, check with your doctor especially if you have dizziness.

A lot of police officers have a pulse between sixty-four and seventy-two, and that's put them in good shape. You see if you are on no meds, not overweight, and active and have a pulse of sixty-four, you have to have a good functioning heart and the lungs are absorbing the oxygen well. The blood is in good level with anemia. A lot of things have to come together to have that nice pulse. This is usually with good BP equals long life if you avoid or escape trauma and tumor.

So if you check your BP and it is 150 over 90, you have mild high BP. If you take meds and it is the same, this means that either the meds are low dose or you are not helping the meds with your diet and weight and drinks. Your doctor will help.

BP is a negative factor. It can kill you in the long run. One of the ways is by increasing the size of the ventricle muscle, and with age, the blood supply is not enough, resulting to myopathy and

Heart Failure

The effect depends on additional negative factors, and on the type of BP, there is prehypertension. There is mild, moderate, and the severe type.

If you want to be more sophisticated, if there is a big difference between the top and bottom pressures like 160 over 70, which is over sixty points, it may be from high thyroid or vascular occlusion in the legs or maybe an increased cardiac output like from anemia.

Check your eyes for the following:

- If it is yellow, it is important to see a doctor now.
- If you hit your head and then you find some blood under the conjunctiva, see a doctor too. It may be coming from the brain.

Check your skin.

If you have a lump or a pump in your body and you can feel it, check with your doctor. It may be a tumor. If the doctor says it is a benign problem and after one year it started bleeding or growing fast or painful, check with your surgeon. Benign lumps can change with time.

Check your temperature.

If your mouth temperature is more than the axillary temperature, you may have thyrotoxicosis (hyperfunctioning of the thyroid).

For a woman, a monthly breast self-exam is essential; feeling a lump is a serious problem. A general surgeon, breast surgeon, and vascular surgeon are good to see.

If you have fever with activity, you may have tuberculosis.

Check your weight.

If you lose weight fast, without dieting, check for diabetes or stomach cancer.

Aging

Decaying of the mitochondria, which is present in the center of the cell. It is the one which can use the fat or sugar to give you energy. It works more efficiently at young age up to three times, so to improve its functions, there are the supplements like the trace elements as zinc and manganese and vitamins to help the mitochondria do its job better.

Alzheimer's disease

Part of it is memory loss. Now if you forget where you put your glasses, it is okay, but if you forget that you have glasses, you better find help.

It is Alzheimer's when there is decline in the intellectual function secondary to a degenerative disorder in which old information can't be reached, and new ones can't be stored. The brain is covered with plaques, which interfere with the neurons' communications. The area of memory is called the hippocampus in the brain. Other causes include multiple small strokes, late syphilis, and brain tumors, as well as deposits of aluminum in the hippocampus and aluminum in water. Antacids may be the cause of Alzheimer's in a high number of cases.

Aluminum is in the soil, air, water, and small amounts in food. It is also present in aluminum cooking wares, cooking utensils, and foil. Since it is in antacids and it is used in large amounts by people, it is probably the highest reason for its toxicity like Maalox and Mylanta exrastrength, Amphogel, Gaviscan tab or liquid has it; but Alka-Seltzer, Tums, Rolaids, Maalox, and Mylanta gel caps and regular strength liquid do not have it.

Also, it is in antidiarrhea, Donnagel, Kaopectate aluminum magnesium silicate, pepto besmol and rheopan, buffered ascriptin and aspirin with antacid, deodorants, and douches.

To Reduce Aluminum Toxicity

Aluminum absorption increases by acidic foods—coffee, tea, tomato, meats; but apple pectin absorbs the toxins and removes it with the stool.

B complex vitamins—B6 and B12 detoxifies toxic metals in the intestine.

We can also use garlic.

Use stainless steel and glassware.

Chelation therapy but not for Alzheimer's.

The deeper you cook, the more aluminum is in your food.

Diagnosis

Hair Analysis

- Food additive in frozen foods, pickles, tartar, cheeseburgers, and processed cheese.
- Aluminum is added to give foods melting quality.

Differential Diagnoses

Rule out low thyroid, brain tumors, Vitamin B12 deficiency, low zinc. Decrease the growth of the neurofibrillary connecting nerve cells in malabsorption syndrome.

Aluminum toxicity is associated with osteoporosis and kidney disease because it is excreted there. It is also seen in Alzheimer's disease.

The crusts are beta-amyloid present in other areas in the body; it is a sort of cell decay, but it is high in Alzheimer's.

Few millions in the USA have it. It mostly starts at sixty-five but can be earlier, and 50 percent of people over eighty years has it. It is a serious disease. It is a progressive, disabling disease; it invites falls, fractures, accidents. It kills one hundred thousand per year.

Nutrition:

Apple pectin
L-carnitine
300 mg acetylcholine per day
3 mg Boron
Flaxseed
100 mg CoQ10
Ginkgo biloba
Multivitamins
Zinc
Antioxidants, flavonoids

Medications

Most meds have problems, and it is disabling sometimes. For example, if you take one gram of Tylenol four times a day for few weeks, you may develop liver failure. I am talking about the largest organ in your body, which detoxifies most metabolized products, including meds. By the way, Tylenol is one of the safest, most used drugs in meds, but you have to know how much to take and how long or you will pay if you take more than 1,000 mg four times a day for two weeks. The biggest organ in your body can fail and give severe complications.

Aspirin Complications

These can give you bleeding in the stomach even from the first pill. The bleeding may be massive. By the way, aspirin works on the stomach in two ways. One is localized if you take it by mouth, and the other, after it reaches, it affects the stomach mucus lining and the acid production. The larger the dose the worse.

Simple aspirin may increase bleeding in the brain or eyes and gives disability, especially with blood thinners like Coumadin.

Omega-3 is a very good supplement. If taken with a fat-soluble good dose vitamin A, can ake vit a toxic.

Cortisone

For side effects, never forget it. This one is not a game.

If it is given in injection form, in a good dose, this may result to depression and suicidal problem. A patient jumped from the third floor, fractured her hip but survived. You will ask how she can jump. Yes, the windows were easy to raise before the accident.

For asthma, cortisone is given daily for long periods. Please watch the asthmatics from the above complications.

Eyedrops

One drop of Alphagan can give you somnolence. Like in sleeping, even though you know you need to breath, but you can't. This is called sleep apnea. Or you just sit on a sofa. A patient told me he will go to sleep and hit the desk with his head, and he did not know why. I tell you if he was in a car driving, he could be in trouble.

A simple Benadryl tablet can do the same. It is over the counter. It comes in 25 mg. Don't drive with it.

Narcotics, alcoholics, you know by now that driving with this is deadly for you and the one who is with you or in front of your car.

You have to read or let someone read it for you. The pharmacy gives you a lot of information about reactions and side effects.

Other Factors

Do you have any negative factors like high blood pressure and high cholesterol? Smoking, you are at a higher risk if you don't get help.

Chapter 11

Osteoporosis

Osteoporosis is a progressive disease in which the loss of minerals, primarily calcium, causes bones to become more and more fragile. Its name refers to the "pores" or tiny holes in bone. Hypnosis, loss of height, and fractures of the ankle, wrist, hip, and spine often occur in people with severe osteoporosis; and the disease is more common in women than men. Osteoporosis can be disabling and deadly, and it must be prevented.

Bone Mass

Bone mass, which is the amount of minerals in bones, is highest at thirty to thirty-five years of age and decreases by 35 percent between the ages of fifty and seventy years. A lack of calcium is not the only cause of osteoporosis. Other contributing factors include the following conditions:

- A deficiency in vitamins A, C, D, E, or K
- A deficiency in magnesium, phosphorous, boron, zinc or copper
- Estrogen deficiency
- Lack of exercise
- A high-sugar diet

- Poor calcium absorption caused by a bowel disease
- Menopause
- Heavy consumption of coffee, tea, or alcohol
- Endocrine disease, such as a high level of parathyroid hormone.
- Cortisone therapy, even for just a few weeks

Remember these facts:

- Asians have a higher incidence of osteoporosis than Americans do.
- African-Americans have a lower incidence of osteoporosis than do white Americans.
- People with a large frame have a relatively lower incidence of osteoporosis.
- Underweight people older than seventy years are more prone to hip fracture (unless they have strong bones) than are people of the same age whose weight is within the normal range because thin people have no cushion of fat to protect their hips during a fall.

Eight million women and two million men in America have osteoporosis, and that disorder is becoming more prevalent. In addition, thirty million Americans have osteopenia, which is an early stage of bone thinning. Fewer men than women have osteoporosis. Women should begin their annual checkups for bone thinning at the age of forty-five years, and men should do so at the age of sixty-five years. Osteoporosis develops in 30 to 40 percent of women and 10 to 12 percent of men older than fifty years. Fifty percent of women older than fifty-five years have low bone mass. Each year in America, there are fifty thousand cases of fractures of the spine that are caused by coughing or sneezing vigorously. Those fractures are disabling, and they can be deadly if they are complicated by a pulmonary embolus—a blood clot in the lungs. Each year in America, 30 percent of people with a fracture of the hip from a subsequent pulmonary embolus die within three to six months of the fracture.

Bone Strength

Bone strength equals bone quantity, which depends on the bone density and frame size, plus bone quality or the strength of the matrix or architecture of the bone. It needs a biopsy to know its value, and it is not usually done.

Bone density depends on the quantity of calcium in the bones, which can be measured. When bony material is lost, bones become thin and change shape. Kyphosis usually develops, and a person with that condition can lose up to three inches in height. The most common sites of fracture in an osteoporotic person are the spine (a compression fracture)—most common site is eleventh vertebra, the wrist, and the hip and/or pelvis.

Of those types, fractures of the hip and spine are the worst. They are disabling, and they can result in a poor quality of life or even death. Osteoporosis is a silent disease. It is the most common cause of spine fracture, which is most likely to occur in tenth, eleventh, or twelfth thoracic vertebra. The most common type of fracture is the compression fracture. Millions of people today are unaware that they have low bone density. A woman older than fifty years has a 40 percent chance in her lifetime of having an osteoporotic problem. Of osteoporotic women older than sixty-five years, 25 percent will have a chronic deformity, and 15 percent of those with a fracture will be permanently disabled.

A DEXA scan for one hundred dollars can diagnose the thinning, and there is a lot of good available medications, which can stop or at least decrease the incidence these type of disabling fractures. What I am trying to say is that people who have cancer die months or years from the cancer, but people who have osteoporosis get disabled and die within few months from a minor fall. This should not be tolerated.

Bone Mineral Density (BMD)

Dual energy X-ray absorptiometry (DEXA), which is safe and accurate, measures bone mineral density (BMD) and reveals bone thinning. The scan is a painless fifteen-minute procedure that can be read on the spot. Two devices are used to perform a DEXA scan, which involves the use of ionizing radiation (it is low, 10 percent of the radiation exposure from a chest radiograph). And ultrasonography is useful for measuring the BMD of the wrists and ankles (I don't recommend since rarely somebody die from fracture of the wrist or ankle), but its results must be confirmed by a DEXA scan. DEXA findings are rated according to BMD on the following scale:

- If your BMD is less than minus 2.5 (-2.5), then you have osteoporosis. You need special medications which will be discussed later, plus calcium, vitamin D, magnesium, boron, copper, and zinc.
- If your BMD is higher than minus 1 (-1 to 4), then you do not have osteoporosis.
- If your BMD is less than—1 to—2.4, then you have osteopenia (early bone thinning). Exercise, high calcium, and minerals may do the job. A second test is to be done in six months.

Pelvic Fractures

In the United States each year, one in every ten thousand people younger than sixty-five years and three people older than that age sustain a fracture. That rate is high. Most fractures that occur in the young people result from trauma, and osteoporosis is the most common cause of fractures in the elderly.

Fracture of the Femur Shaft

A fracture of the femur shaft can cause the rapid transit of a fatty embolus to the lungs, which results in pulmonary insufficiency. However, a blood clot in the legs or an embolus of the lungs can also develop a few days after a fracture and can cause sudden death if resuscitation fails. Why fractures of the hip, pelvis, or spine are more serious than other fractures are? Why do 30 percent of the individuals who experience any of those types of fracture die within six months? Factures of the hip, pelvis, or spine require immobilization, which causes many health problems such as a blood clot that blocks the veins of the calf, thigh, or pelvis or that travels to the lungs (a pulmonary embolus) and causes severe respiratory problems or death.

For that reason, a filter can be inserted through a vein in the upper thigh into the inferior vena cava, which is a large vein in the abdomen that transports the embolus directly to the heart, and then it continues from the heart to the lungs. In seconds, it can give a sudden death. That procedure is lifesaving, and the patient requires only a local anesthetic. Patients at risk for blood clots are often treated with a blood-thinning agent if they have no internal bleeding, such as that resulting from a gastric ulcer.

Pneumonia caused by immobility, especially in smokers, those with a chronic lung disorder or heart disease, and the elderly. Immobilized patients are also at risk for the formation of decubitus ulcers (bedsores), which can develop despite the patient's being periodically moved while bedbound. Decubitus ulcers can cause sepsis of the blood, an infection that can usually be controlled.

Thin or Fat: Which Is Better for Your Bones?

Is being thin likely to decrease your risk for hip fracture? A person who weighs less than 125 lb and is five feet four inches tall is thin. However, if you fit that description and you are older than sixty-five years, then weighing ten pounds more is okay because the extra weight will cushion your hips and only a high-power injury will cause a fracture. Protection against fracture may be the only advantage of being heavier rather than thinner; a thin person is more susceptible to fractures caused by trauma. Whether you are thin or heavy, avoid falling. Thin people live longer if they avoid hip, spine, and pelvic injury.

Which Is More Serious: A Fracture of the Hip or Lower Back?

Fractures of the hip or lower back are severe injuries. The incidence of both those fractures has increased in the United States during the past few years, especially in those older than sixty-five years (a population that is increasing because of improvements in the treatment of stroke, heart attack, and cancer). To those who are frail, however, a fall can cause a fracture. According to the Centers for Disease Control and Prevention (CDC), fractures are the second most common cause of death in the United States. American men, in whom the incidence of fracture has increased from thirty-two per one hundred thousand to forty-six per one hundred thousand now sustain more fractures than do American women. If you visit a nursing home, you will notice many wheelchair-bound patients who have sustained a fracture of the hip, back, or spine that may be complicated by leg paralysis. However, if a patient with a fracture of the hip can escape complications, he or she will be walking in few months.

Who Are at Risk for Fracture?

People with any of the following characteristics are at risk for fracture:

Age older than forty-five years in women and sixty-five years in men, although fractures can also occur in younger individuals who have a chronic disease or experience trauma.

A sedentary lifestyle. Exercise strengthens bones and enlarges muscles, but a sedentary lifestyle does the opposite.

Smoking, which has no beneficial effects whatsoever. Even smoking the hubble-bubble or shisha causes osteoporosis because the tobacco smoke is wrapped in aluminum foil. When heat is released, the aluminum in the foil is inhaled, leaching the calcium from bones and causes osteoporosis. At the same time it can start Alzheimer's disease.

Recurrent falls or too-strenuous exercise for your age and fitness level.

Poor muscle tone and a thin body type in Asians and whites.

A family history of osteoporotic fracture.

Car accidents followed by inactivity.

Being thin (e.g., weighing less than 125 lb if you are five feet four inches tall) because thin people have no cushion of fat to protect them when they fall.

A low-calcium, low-magnesium diet.

Little exposure to the sun (low vitamin D).

A low level of vitamin D (low vitamin D diet).

Poor vision (especially night blindness) or legal blindness, which can result in a fall.

Retinopathy—for example, cystoid macular edema. If you have that type of eye disease, be careful on stairs unless you know exactly where and how high each step is. Also, be very cautious when you move from a lighted area to a dim area.

Osteoarthritis and joint disease, especially in poorly nourished individuals.

Thyroid replacement therapy.

Anticonvulsant therapy.

Parathyroid disease. Parathyroid hormone is important to the deposition of calcium in bones. If the level of parathyroid hormone is high, then the level of calcium in the bloodstream will also be high. That extra calcium is extracted from bones, which then become weakened and more susceptible to fracture.

A high salt and phosphate diet. Calcium is excreted in the urine to keep the blood alkaline, resulting to osteoporosis.

Cortisone therapy. If you are treated with oral cortisone for weeks or months, then your risk for osteoporosis, diabetes, obesity, leg edema, and high blood pressure increases.

Bone diseases (such as cancer of bone marrow) requiring treatment with chemotherapy that causes anorexia.

Alcoholism, which results in liver disease and a poor nutritional state.

Poor absorption of nutrients, which can occur as a result of aging or after small bowel surgery.

Anorexia caused by a desire to be fashionable. That type of anorexia, which develops most often in women, can result in muscle disorders and illnesses caused by poor nutrition.

Treatment with an antireflux medication. You Young, MD, from Pennsylvania University, reviewed many patients who were treated with an antireflux medication for one year and found in that group a 40 percent increase in the incidence of osteoporotic fractures. Antireflux drugs decrease the amount of gastric acid in the stomach, which in turn reduces the absorption of calcium. If you are treated with an antireflux medication, take extra calcium (good sources of which are fortified soybeans, cereals, and juices).

Drinking more than four cups of coffee daily, which can cause frequent urination and high blood acidity (both of which leaches calcium, magnesium from bones and the bloodstream).

Vitamin K deficiency.

Avoiding Fractures

Start with a checkup. Research has shown that in 80 percent of individuals who felt well and had no symptoms of osteoporosis, the results of a DEXA scan revealed that disorder. If you do have osteoporosis, then take note of the following:

- Avoid walking on bumpy terrain.
- Avoid exercising too vigorously although exercises that are appropriate for your age and fitness level are beneficial. Building and maintaining a strong healthy body are the most

important factors in preventing fractures because strong muscles and bones resist injury.

- Fix the carpet edges in your home.
- Be careful on slippery stairs.
- Correct poor vision to the greatest extent possible. Remember that the cataract is a conquered disorder!
- Take a daily multivitamin (for example, Centrum, Protegra, or Ocuvite) that contains vitamins A, C, and E as well as selenium and zinc.
- If you have Parkinson's disease and tend to fall frequently, wear a hip-protection shield.
- Eat foods that are high in calcium.

Vitamins

A diet rich in essential vitamins and minerals helps to build strong bones as well as overall good health. Remember these facts about the vitamins that you need each day to ensure the health and strength of your bones:

Vitamin D and sun exposure are necessary for strong bones, but too much sun exposure can cause eye disorders and skin problems.

Be sure that your diet is high in calcium and magnesium.

Consume sufficient quantities of dairy products such as skim milk and low-fat cheese.

Avoid ingesting too much vitamin A. More than 5,000 IU of that vitamin can be toxic and may cause osteoporosis. However, taking beta-carotene as a dietary supplement has no effect on osteoporosis.

Drinking more than four cups of coffee increases urination and calcium loss.

A high-protein diet causes the increased production of acid (the protein end products) that leaches the calcium from blood and bones.

Hypocalcemia

If you suspect that you have hypocalcaemia—a low level of calcium in the blood, then take note of the following:

- Ask your doctor for a blood test that will reveal your calcium level.
- A very high or low level of calcium in the blood is an urgent problem.
- Too little calcium in the bloodstream can cause seizures, tremors, and cardiac emergencies.

If You Have Osteoporosis

If your doctor finds that you have osteoporosis, be sure that each day your diet includes foods that contain calcium such as dairy products and meat and fruits and vegetables, which contain less calcium than that in dairy products and meat or calcium citrate 1,200 to 1,500 per day. Intake of no more than 3 mg of boron, 500 to 750 mg of magnesium, 3 mg of copper, 1 mg of manganese per day, 50 mcg of chromium per day, especially if you have diabetes. Add vitamins A, B, C, E, K (a multivitamin like Centrum or Strovite is okay. Vitamin D 400 C and 100 mcg of vitamin B12 per day.

Exercise

Weight-bearing exercises are beneficial because when a muscle pulls on the bone to which it is attached, it facilitates the deposition of calcium in that bone, which then becomes stronger. Walking a mile each day enables the deposition of a calcium reserve in bone that lasts up to seven years. Although nonweight-bearing exercises are good for the muscles and benefit the bones, weight-bearing exercises produce better results. If you want to prevent or manage osteoporosis, remember these tips:

Do not perform strenuous exercises; walking on a smooth flat surface is sufficient.

Stop smoking and drinking alcohol.

Prevent falls that could occur in the bathtub. Falling in the tub often causes a fracture or an injury to the shoulder and rotator cuff. Place a rubber mat near the tub and don't walk on wet floors.

Some medications (progesterone, phenytoin [Dilantin]) can cause osteoporosis, so you may have to change your treatment regimen and begin to take medications that increase the deposition of calcium in your bones. Drugs that inhibit calcium loss rather than build calcium deposits include alendronate sodium (Fosamax) in tablets (5 or 10 mg daily; 35 or 70 mg per week) or as a syrup. However, Fosamax can cause problems such as gastroesophageal reflux disease or kidney stones, and it must be fortified with vitamin D.

Diet and Supplements

Before you change your diet or begin taking any supplement, ask your doctor for a comprehensive physical examination and a blood test to rule out a tumor, anemia, liver disease, kidney disease, diabetes, calcium in your urine, and Human Immunodeficiency Virus (HIV).

And to determine your levels of thyroid hormone, vitamin D (which should be higher than 30 IU), folate, vitamin B12, and cholesterol.

Preventing and Inhibiting Osteoporosis

Reduce your consumption of or stop drinking soft drinks, which contain phosphoric acid and sugar, both of which are acidic to keep the blood normal and with alkaline pH. The body uses the calcium to neutralize the excess acid produced by the phosphorous and the sugar end products.

Reduce your consumption of drinks that are high in caffeine. Those beverages reduce the absorption of calcium, which is excreted in urine.

Avoid eating a diet high in meat, especially if you have bone thinning. Meat, when digested and absorbed into the bloodstream, is acidic. Calcium is lost when it neutralizes that acid.

Be sure that you do not have an imbalance in your levels of parathyroid hormone (which stimulates cells called *osteoclasts* to remove calcium from bones) or low level of the thyroid hormone which stimulates the osteoblasts, the calcium builders calcitonin. An excessively high level of parathyroid hormone (hyperparathyroidism) or low calcitonin can precede the development of osteoporosis.

Eat alkaline foods such as fruits, vegetables, juices, and buckwheat.

Other grains like those used to make alcoholic beverages are acidic.

Eat a diet that is high in calcium, magnesium, and manganese.

Perform weight-bearing exercises three times a week, no strenuous exercises period, weights, and see a doctor first.

Decrease your stress level.

Avoid treatment with cortisone or shorten the duration of treatment.

Consume enough vitamin C, which increases calcium absorption.

Consume enough vitamin D and get enough exposure to the sun.

Consume enough vitamin K, which is found in green vegetables.

Reducing Your Risk for Osteoporosis

Be sure to ingest enough calcium and magnesium as described above. The amount of calcium in the bloodstream depends on your body's ability to absorb that mineral, which is influenced by your age, the amount of calcium consumed, and the condition of your intestines. Calcium is essential for the normal growth and development of children because 90 percent of bone mass is formed before the age of twenty years. To build strong and healthy bones, add calcium, magnesium, vitamin D, fruits, and vegetables to your daily diet and exercise to your daily routine.

Why is magnesium essential? A low-magnesium diet (even when coupled with a high calcium intake) will not prevent osteoporosis. That ratio is ten to one. Usually it has to be three is to one.

Sources of Calcium: Diet or Supplements?

Calcium can be consumed in foods like cheese and beverages such as milk, or it can be ingested in a supplement. Let's examine those sources of calcium in greater detail.

Dietary sources of calcium

Foods high in calcium include the following:

> 1 cup of goat milk (the highest in calcium of all types of milk): 300 to 500 mg of calcium.
> 1 cup of whole (cow) milk: 300 mg
> 1 cup of skim (cow) milk: 300 mg
> One cup soy milk fortified 400 mg
> 3 oz canned fish with bones: 250 mg
> 3 oz of sardines: 250 mg
> 1 oz of cheddar cheese: 200 mg
> 1 oz of Swiss cheese: 250 mg
> 1 oz of cottage cheese: 150 mg
> 1 oz of mozzarella cheese: 400 mg

People with lactose intolerance, which is common in blacks, Asians, native Americans, and some people of European descent, can obtain sufficient calcium by adding lactated tablets (over the counter) to "regular" milk, choosing packaged lactose-free milk, eating sardines, taking a calcium supplement, and/or consuming fortified cereals, fortified soybean milk, and juices.

If you have high levels of bad cholesterol, drink low-fat Milk.

- Other sources of calcium
  Quarter cup of sesame seeds 350 mg
  Calcium fortified orange juice 300 mg
  Spinach one cup cooked 300 mg
  Almonds one oz 75 mg
  Orange medium size 50 mg
  One egg 55 mg
  Beans half cup 60 mg

Calcium supplements

Over-the-counter calcium supplements can be purchased in doses of 500 or 1,000 mg, and they usually also contain vitamin D. Here are the recommended daily values of calcium for women and men:

A woman older than fifty-five years 1,500 mg
A pregnant woman 1,500 mg
A woman younger than fifty years 1,000 mg
A woman taking estrogen 1,500 mg
A man older than fifty years 1,000 mg

If your intake of vitamin D is low, you should not begin treatment with Fosamax until your level of that vitamin has been corrected by treatment prescribed by your doctor. Remember that drinking milk to ingest the calcium necessary for bone health is a good idea unless your intake of magnesium is low. Too little magnesium can cause osteoporosis. In milk, the ratio of calcium to magnesium is twenty to one. To build bones, that ratio must be three to one.

Magnesium

Magnesium is an essential mineral that has hundreds of physiologic uses. Chronic alcoholism reduces the level of magnesium in the body. People with a deficiency of magnesium, boron, selenium, and B vitamins are at risk for osteoporosis. The recommended daily value of magnesium is 250 to 500 mg. An over-the-counter drug called calcium, magnesium, and zinc with copper can supply the required daily value of magnesium if taken in a dosage of one and one-half tablets daily. That supplement contains 1,000 mg of calcium, 400 mg of magnesium, 15 mg of zinc, and 1 mg of copper.

In addition to that product, take a daily multivitamin that contains 400 mcg of vitamin D.

Calcium Toxicity

If the level of calcium in your bloodstream is too high, arrhythmia, diarrhea, and dehydration can develop.

Vitamin D

The recommended dose of vitamin D is 400 mcg daily, but if you have a low level of that vitamin in your bloodstream, your doctor may recommend a higher dose. Research has shown that taking calcium with magnesium, phosphate, selenium, and vitamin D will reduce your risk for osteoporosis. People in their forties can ingest an adequate amount of vitamin D by eating two ounces of cheese and drinking one cup of milk, a combination that supplies about

1,000 mcg of that vitamin. Additional vitamin D will be supplied by other foods consumed.

Other Benefits of Calcium

Remember, a diet that is high calcium and potassium and low in salt lowers high blood pressure, decreases the risk for stroke, decreases the risk for rectal cancer, improves fatty acid metabolism, which provides energy and augments weight loss.

Types of Calcium

The best form of supplementary calcium is calcium citrate.

It is weakly acidic and thus enhances calcium absorption, so avoid taking antireflux or antacid medications if you are also taking a calcium supplement. You can take calcium citrate on an empty stomach or before you go to sleep.

Calcium Carbonate

When compared with calcium citrate, calcium carbonate is less well absorbed. Remember the following:

- Don't take a calcium supplement within four hours of having taken a thyroid medication because thyroid medications decrease the absorption of calcium.
- Don't take a calcium supplement if you have a high level of parathyroid hormone (which causes a very high level of calcium in your bloodstream).

- Don't take a calcium supplement if you have a high level of vitamin D in your bloodstream.

Bone Builders

Osteoblasts are cells that build bone, and osteoclasts are cells that remove calcium from bones, which are stimulated by low levels of estrogen and parathyroid hormone and by treatment with cortisone can cause osteoporosis.

Prescription Medications for the Treatment of Osteoporosis

The following medications must be prescribed by a doctor, who must monitor their effects. Remember that some diseases, such as leukemia, sarcoidosis, and lymphoma increase the levels of vitamin D, calcium, and magnesium in the bloodstream.

Risedronate sodium (Actonel), which is taken daily, is available as oral tablets in doses of 5 mg per day or 35 mg once per week. Actonel stops or reverses osteoporosis.

Alendronate sodium (Fosamax), which is taken daily or weekly, is available as oral tablets in doses of 5 or 10 mg per day and 35 to 70 mg per week or as a syrup (one bottle per week). You must sit or stand for thirty minutes after having taken this medication. Avoid taking Fosamax if you have gastric reflux disease, a duodenal or stomach ulcer, a low serum level of calcium, or an allergy to any ingredients in that medication.

Fosamax plus vitamin D.

Ibandronate sodium (Boniva) 2.5 mg daily or 150 mg tablet of which is taken monthly reverses bone loss by stopping calcium loss. If the oral form of that drug cannot be tolerated, then one injection of Boniva can be administered every three months. People with a low level of calcium should not take Boniva.

Note: The medications listed above are effective treatments for osteoporosis, but they can cause nausea and exacerbate stomach ulcers. Patients treated with those agents must undergo regularly scheduled blood tests and urinalysis to monitor their serum levels of liver enzymes, vitamin D, and calcium as well as kidney parameters.

The parathyroid hormone controls the level of calcium in the bloodstream. A high serum level of calcium may indicate a tumor of the parathyroid, and a low level indicates the need for parathyroid hormone replacement.

It is important to remember that if you are taking a medication, you must ensure that your body is adequately nourished. Successful treatment requires vitamins, minerals, and trace elements such as magnesium. When you build bone, you must build collagen, which requires protein. You need energy to produce new body cells, and you also need antioxidants to neutralize the effects of free radicals, which are wastes generated by cell metabolism You need nonstrenuous exercise to strengthen muscles that will protect you if you fall. You need a healthy liver to detoxify the end products of cell metabolism, and you must have healthy kidneys to excrete body waste. Reducing your risk for Alzheimer's disease and osteoporosis depends on sufficient and appropriate exercise and a healthful diet that includes fruits, vegetables, beans, meat, fish, vitamins, calcium, and silicon.

To stop osteoporosis, you need to take calcium, magnesium, manganese, vitamin D, copper, silicon, zinc, and boron.

Calcium alone for osteoporosis is insufficient, so take antioxidants. One pill called Protegra can be taken daily plus another called calcium A plus D and minerals (both are over the counter). Protegra has vitamins A, C, E, selenium, and zinc. The other medicine (OTC)is calcium 600 mg plus D, magnesium, manganese, copper, and zinc. You need one pill twice a day.

Silicon helps with the growth of bones, hair, and skin.

Boron increases absorption of calcium and transforms vitamin D to its active form.

Copper strengthens bones, tendons, and nerves.

Manganese, essential for formation and maintenance of bones.

Zinc is for bone development, bone strength, and growth.

Thanks,
A. Taha

INDEX

G

W